*f*P

BEATING BACK

THE 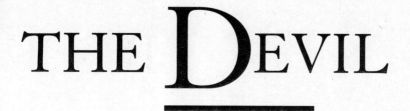DEVIL

ON THE FRONT LINES WITH
THE DISEASE DETECTIVES OF THE
EPIDEMIC INTELLIGENCE SERVICE

MARYN McKENNA

FREE PRESS

NEW YORK   LONDON   TORONTO   SYDNEY

*f*P

FREE PRESS
A Division of Simon & Schuster, Inc.
1230 Avenue of the Americas
New York, NY 10020

FREE PRESS and colophon are trademarks
of Simon & Schuster, Inc.

For information regarding special discounts for bulk purchases,
please contact Simon & Schuster Special Sales at 1-800-456-6798
or business@simonandschuster.com

Designed by Leslie Phillips

Manufactured in the United States of America

10 9 8 7 6 5 4 3 2 1

Library of Congress Cataloging-in-Publication Data

McKenna, Maryn.
Beating back the devil : on the front lines with the disease detectives of
the Epidemic Intelligence Service / Maryn McKenna
p. cm.
Includes bibliographical references and index.
1. Centers for Disease Control (U.S.). Epidemic Intelligence Service—Popular works.
2. Epidemiology—Popular works. 3. Epidemiologists—United States—Popular works.
I. Title.

RA653.M38 2004
614.4—dc22   2004053214

ISBN 0-7432-5132-6

614.4

For John James McKenna,

Mary Joan Lauder McKenna

and Mimi Draffen McKenna,

my parents.

CONCERNING THEMSELVES to enquire about it, in order to be certain of the truth, two Physicians and a Surgeon were order'd to go to the House, and make Inspection. This they did; and finding evident Tokens of the Sickness upon both the Bodies that were dead, they gave their Opinions publicly, that they died of the Plague.

—DANIEL DEFOE, 1722

INFECTIOUS DISEASE is one of the few genuine adventures left in the world.

—HANS ZINSSER, 1934

CONTENTS

CONTENTS

BEATING BACK
THE DEVIL

July 2002, Anniston, Alabama

THE CINDER BLOCK HALLWAY is wide, white, and chilly. Brilliant fluorescent light glares off the slick paint. The light makes pools of brightness on the linoleum, leaving the ends of the corridor in shadow.

In one of the pools of brightness, a body is lying on a gurney.

A crew of health care workers huddles around it. They are shrouded in baggy white coveralls, thick boots, and black rubber gauntlets that reach their elbows. Heavy military respirators mask their faces, tugging down their heads and cutting off their peripheral vision. Their instructor stands at the side of the stretcher; when his voice booms out, the faceplates swivel in his direction like a nervous flock of periscopes.

"Someone has placed a device in a trash container at the food court in the mall," he says. "It contained Sarin gas. Several people have collapsed. This is one of them."

The Tyvek suits crinkle as the workers crowd the gurney. They are anxious in the unfamiliar surroundings, nervous about the task in front of them, eager to get started treating their patient. Their instructor knows this. He knows they have been taught to move quickly and decisively. He also knows, as they will learn, how much danger their rapid reflexes could put them in now.

"Your training is to get the patient to treatment as soon as possible," he says. "But you need to cut his clothes off first. You need to wipe him down with decontaminant. If you rush into the emergency room with this person, you may create a bigger problem than you already have. People in that emergency room may die because of you."

Clutching sponges, four of the health workers crouch awkwardly by the stretcher, taking care not to kneel and contaminate the fragile suits that protect them from poison-gas residue. One eases off the patient's shoes. Two cut carefully through his clothing with scissors, pulling the cloth away from his skin. The fourth, at the head of the stretcher, monitors the victim's vital signs.

Or would, if he had any. The victim's chest is not rising. The fingers seeking a pulse make no dent on his plastic skin. The body on the gurney is a training dummy, a jointed plastic mannequin wearing thrift-shop clothes and a synthetic wig that the sponges have knocked askew.

It looks like a joke figure, something to stuff in a porch rocking chair on Halloween, but there is nothing light-hearted about this training session. Instead, it is tense and solemn. It represents the first time in more than fifty years that the U.S. government has prepared its disease detectives for an ugly possibility: that the health problems they will be chasing may be deliberately caused.

The members of the group around the gurney are the newest enrollees in the Epidemic Intelligence Service of the U.S. Centers for Disease Control and Prevention. The CDC is the Pentagon of public health in America, the place where threats are identified and control strategies are launched. The EIS is its Special Forces.

The members of the disease detective corps have always been young, highly trained, and fiercely committed. They expect to be summoned in the middle of the night for a crisis halfway across the country, or the world. But they have never before been trained to be the first responders to radioactive, chemical, and biological attacks.

The EIS was founded in 1951 because health authorities feared Korean War troops had been exposed to biological weapons. The fear was groundless, then. Fifty-one years later, bioweapons have not yet been used against U.S. troops—but they have been against U.S. civilians. It is reasonable to believe they will be used again.

It is ten months since two hijacked planes brought down New York City's World Trade Center, and nine months since a set of mailed envelopes, loaded with finely milled anthrax, accomplished the first fatal bioterrorist attack in American history on American soil. The eighty-nine doctors, Ph.D.s, veterinarians, and nurses in this EIS class applied for their jobs before the World Trade Center was attacked. They were offered their positions, and accepted them, months afterward—with the understanding that preparing for the possibility of terrorism would be part of the job from now on.

"We can't prevent a terrorist attack," the instructor says. "But we can be better prepared. If you respond properly, you may save a lot of lives, including your own."

But it was one thing to agree to be prepared and another to experience it. It is difficult to move in the billowy suits, and impossible to laugh or catch someone else's eye through the tunnel vision of the faceplate. The loose boots make it hard to walk and impossible to run, even with a drill instructor shouting at their shoulder blades. One of the doctors is clenching his fist to control his anxiety; another is breathing deeply to keep her rising claustrophobia under control.

They have been on the job for three weeks.

Over the instructor's shoulder, a window set into a door offers a glimpse of a disaster scene: a restaurant patio strewn with bodies. Through a second door, there is a second disaster scene: a subway platform, eerily deserted. Both rooms are stage sets, meant to provide practice in the possible varieties of disaster. They serve as a warning: The EIS officers must be prepared to combat terrorism, but they cannot predict where or how it will appear.

Behind this training session lies an assumption: There will be another terrorist attack, of some kind, and the EIS will be the ones who respond to it. They will have to calm panicked citizens, rally dazed medical personnel, and organize care of the victims. They will be the most knowledgeable people on the scene of a disaster, and they will have to take charge for the first few hours—or, if things go very badly, for the first few days.

Until that happens, they will take up the daily jobs of disease detectives, racing to health problems that range from small clusters of food-borne illness to nationwide outbreaks of newly discovered pathogens. But first they will spend a week in this disused Army hospital, learning to rush toward threats that any sensible human would run from.

"I cannot emphasize this enough: You are a target, a target, a target," their trainer tells them. "If they take you out, there will be no one to hold the line on whatever epidemic they have caused."

ONE

Training
July 2002, Atlanta

ON A HUMID, SUNNY MORNING in July 2002, a group of eighty-nine men and women met in a windowless auditorium in an unremarkable pale-brick building set in a leafy suburban neighborhood in northeast Atlanta.

The building, the street-side face of a sprawling warren of cubicles, laboratories, and conference rooms, was the headquarters of the U.S. Centers for Disease Control and Prevention, usually known as the CDC. The CDC is the public health agency for the federal government, the organization charged with identifying, tracking, and trying to prevent the infectious and chronic diseases, environmental hazards, and workplace dangers that may afflict Americans.

At least, that was its official mission. Over its fifty-six years of existence, the CDC's duties—and even more, its reputation—had outgrown that dry description. Within its undistinguished 1960s-style architecture, made interesting only by a small marble bust of Hygieia, the Greek goddess of health, in front of the building and some expensive new laboratories rising behind it, worked people who were responsible for eradicating smallpox, the world's worst killer. Its scientists had identified Legionnaires' disease and hantavirus pulmonary syndrome, and had come face to face with Ebola virus and survived. Its researchers had taught Third World villagers low-cost, low-tech ways to protect their drinking water from terrifying parasites. Its acronym was recognized around the globe, often by people who had no idea what its initials meant.

On the inside, the CDC was a combination of cumbersome bureaucracy, research university, idealistic nonprofit, and skunk works. From the outside, it had acquired an unlikely glamour. Imagined versions of its researchers had been featured in movies and best-selling novels—usually, to its employees' sour amusement, in far more plush surroundings than the ones they actually worked in.

The group waiting in the auditorium on that hot July morning was feeling far from glamorous. Its members were variously nervous, excited, jet-lagged, grumpily undercaffeinated, appalled by the heat, anxious over a baby just dropped off for her first-ever morning of day care, and wondering with a thrill of apprehension what they had gotten themselves into.

They were the newest cadre of recruits to the Epidemic Intelligence Service, the fifty-first entering class of the CDC's rapid-reaction force. They had agreed to trade two years of their careers for two years of intensive training in real-time disease detection. They had accepted, along with the training, a commitment to leave at a moment's notice for whatever outbreak needed them, whether it was a deadly new encephalitis on the far side of the planet or a church-supper attack of diarrhea one state away.

This was their first day.

At the front of the auditorium, Polly Marchbanks, a silver-haired nurse and Ph.D. in a rainbow-striped dress, looked out at the recruits.

"I advise you to fasten your seatbelts," she said. "This is going to be difficult."

In the group that assembled in Atlanta that morning—the class of 2002, named by a quirk of CDC tradition for the year they enrolled rather than the year they would graduate—there were thirty-two men and fifty-seven women; seventy-five Americans and fourteen from other countries; sixty-three Caucasians, fourteen Asians, nine of African heritage, and three whose background was Spanish-speaking.

The EIS is a corps of health professionals; it accepts doctors, dentists, Ph.D.s in some disciplines, physicians' assistants, nurses, and veterinarians. The class of 2002 included fifty-six physicians, twenty-three Ph.D.s, seven veterinarians, two nurses, a dentist, and, for the first time, a lawyer. Each of them, to get their slot, had succeeded over at least two other applicants. Seven of them were Phi Beta Kappa members. Six had been college athletes and four were former Peace Corps volunteers. More than half of them were married or partnered. One was pregnant. Nine of them had children who were not yet walking.

The signature tool of the EIS is epidemiology, the quantitative study of the distribution of disease in populations. Epidemiologists count cases of disease, discern whether there are trends, and devise strategies if the trends need to be reversed. Health workers' exposure to epidemiology varies with their professional training. A Ph.D. in biostatistics might be steeped in it. A family-practice physician might have taken one course in epidemiology early in medical school, and by the time he was done with residency, have forgotten everything he learned five years earlier.

To make sure all its recruits know as much epidemiology as they need to, the CDC puts its new EIS members through what it politely calls a refresher. For three weeks, the group would cram the basics of finding cases, designing studies, and handling lab samples. In effect, they were beginning with boot camp: Epi 101, sixteen hours a day.

"When you arrive at an outbreak, you will find that you get very different reactions to your arrival," said Doug Hamilton, the EIS's chief. A tall, genial family physician and microbiologist who frequently wore Hawaiian shirts to the office, he had headed the EIS for five years. He was born the week the corps was founded, and joined it in 1991 after meeting an EIS member at his twentieth high school reunion. "You will get everything from, 'This is my investigation, back off,' to, 'Thank God, the cavalry has arrived.'"

The new EIS members had been assigned seats in the auditorium at cafeteria-style tables arranged across its width. The seating was alphabetical by last name. It was an uncomplicated method for imposing order on a group that was wildly diverse.

In the front row sat Karen Broder, a pediatrician from a medical family—her father had been director of the National Cancer Institute—who had left private practice to join the EIS. She and her husband, an assistant professor at Emory University next door to the CDC, had two sons, who were three and a half and five years old. She had been pregnant with the younger boy while she was a resident at Massachusetts General Hospital in Boston; she joked that the first noises he recognized were her voice and the sound of her beeper.

Near her sat Wayne Duffus, a Jamaican-born physician and virologist whose family had emigrated to the Bronx when he was in high school. Duffus, who published his first scientific paper when he was still a teenager, had spent all of his academic career in New York City: bachelor's degree from Brooklyn College, M.D. and Ph.D. from Albert Einstein College of Medicine, residency at Columbia-Presbyterian Hospital. For the past year, he had been an infectious diseases fellow at Emory, concentrating on HIV. He had always been torn between the broad implications of lab research and the fine details of patient care; he hoped that coming to the CDC, with its focus on the health of groups, would let him find a middle ground.

Next to him sat Danice Eaton, a Ph.D. in behavioral science who had been an AmeriCorps volunteer, and Kirsten Ernst, a nurse with two master's degrees. Behind them—but not sitting together, because changing seats was frowned on—were Scott Filler and Sami Gottlieb, both doctors and the only married couple in the class. Gottlieb, an internist, had wanted to be an EIS officer since she finished medical school. Meeting Scott, who was three years younger in age but six years behind her in training, had put the goal on hold until he finished as well. They had just returned from volunteering for the summer at an AIDS program in Vietnam.

In between them was Victoria Gammino, an anthropologist with a Ph.D. in international health who had done her dissertation on tuberculosis on a remote atoll in the Pacific, part of the Marshall Islands. Close by sat Alexandre Macedo de Oliveira, an infectious-disease specialist from São Paulo, Brazil, who had applied three times to get into the EIS, and Angela McGowan, the corps' first lawyer. She was a second-generation EIS officer; she had been born during her father's EIS assignment thirty-one years earlier. Her father and her mother both still worked in public health. She had resisted the family business as long as she could, studying international relations in college and international law afterward, but then she succumbed and went for a public health degree as well.

In the same row was Joel Montgomery, a microbiologist from Texas who had already worked at the CDC for two years as a postdoc in parasitic diseases. He was also, as far as anyone knew, the only one in the group to have been in a movie. While working on his Ph.D., he had been caught on camera by a documentary crew filming Komodo dragons—poisonous, eight-foot-long reptiles—in Indonesia. Komodo dragons kill their prey by chewing on them and leaving mouth bacteria in the wound; the prey dies of blood poisoning several days later, and the dragons eat the carcass. Montgomery had been after the same bacteria. He had swabbed the mouths of the thrashing, angry animals while five Indonesian assistants held the reptiles down. After fifteen years in lab science, he was eager to come out from behind the bench, to study the human impact of disease.

In the back of the auditorium were Jennifer Gordon Wright, a veterinarian who had had her first child, a daughter, two months earlier, and John Watson, a South Carolina native who had worked as a family practitioner in Alaska and Seattle and gotten a public-health degree in London. He had wanted to apply to the EIS since he had visited a friend working at the CDC eight years before. His years caring for patients, many of them low-income, had left him with a deep political commitment to health care as a basic right. At the CDC, which had sent two generations of epidemiologists fanning across the globe to improve the health of distant countries, he thought his views would find a home.

The CDC had humble beginnings: It started in 1942 as a government bureau called the Office of Malaria Control in War Areas. "War areas" took in most of the southern states, where there were dozens of military bases to train troops being sent to World War II and hundreds of industrial establishments—boatyards, airfields, factories, and shipping depots—working to support the war effort. Mosquito-borne diseases were a severe challenge for the coastal United States, especially in the South. In the summer of 1853, yellow fever killed more than nine thousand people just in New Orleans; throughout the nineteenth century, yellow-fever quarantines had routinely closed southern port cities. The debilitating recurrent fever of malaria was such a constant in southern life that it had fueled the colonial-era slave trade. European indentured servants sickened and died of malaria; searching for replacements, planters realized that West Africans who had been exposed to malaria since childhood appeared to have some immunity against the disease. In 1942, malaria still persisted in more than thirty states.

Mosquito-borne diseases historically had troubled the military as well, so much so that the U.S. Army funded the research that in 1900 determined mosquitoes were responsible for transmitting yellow fever. Money for the antimalarial drug quinine was one of the first military expenditures authorized by the Continental Congress in the Revolutionary War. Malaria in military personnel had been a persistent and intractable problem ever since.

Malaria control meant, essentially, mosquito control, which before the U.S. patent for DDT was issued in 1943 required searching out the swamps, ditches, and stagnant ponds where mosquito larvae were maturing and either clearing the water of pests with insecticide or smothering the larvae on the surface of the water with oil. DDT made the process much simpler. It killed mosquito adults as well as larvae, so it could be used where the insects encountered humans instead of only where they bred, and once it was sprayed on a surface its effects lasted a long time. Still, DDT's success created more work for the Office of Malaria Control, rather than less. The new chemical was so effective and so cheap that it stimulated wider demand for mosquito control and led to a national program, created by Congress in 1945, that offered to spray civilian homes and businesses as well.

The moquito programs quickly built the Office of Malaria Control in War Areas into a sizable government unit. It had a significant budget and training facilities and laboratories in several states, as well as fleets of trucks and several thousand employees to handle the labor-intensive jobs of mosquito control. But it was also a wartime creation with a limited mandate. That left its parent agency, the U.S. Public Health Service, wondering what to do with the new bureau and its possessions once the war ended. The solution, suggested by an assistant surgeon general named Joseph W. Mountin, was to make the malaria-control unit into a peacetime health agency. It would handle diseases caused by insects and parasites, and expand into tracking other infectious diseases as well. Congress approved the change in 1946; it dubbed the new agency the Communicable Disease Center, giving it initials that would persist through three name changes and come to be recognized worldwide.

The Public Health Service was the original federal health agency: It had been chartered by Congress in 1798 to operate public hospitals for sailors. Over 150 years it had grown to take in quarantine offices at ports, immigrant examination stations such as Ellis Island, venereal disease eradication campaigns, field teams of health investigators who tackled rural problems such as hookworm and trachoma, hospitals for military veterans, and research laboratories. Mountin headed a Health Service division called the Bureau of State Services that forged links between the federal agency and state health departments. He intended the new CDC to strengthen those links, funneling assistance and eventually money to the states.

Giving assistance to the states implied going out into the field to find and control disease outbreaks—effectively the same task the agency had performed for malaria control, but expanded to include other diseases. The mission made the new CDC the mirror image of the sixteen-year-old National Institute (later Institutes) of Health, which began as the National Hygienic Laboratory and conducted basic research into infectious and chronic diseases. Lab research was the heart of NIH's work. But at the CDC, which had built up its laboratories in order to do malaria research, Mountin envisioned the labs not as the center of the agency but as support for the work its personnel were doing with state health departments.

Despite the difference in mission there was conflict between the two agencies. Scientists at NIH and its predecessors had investigated outbreaks as well, though usually in support of an existing research program—that is, not to respond to the emergency, but because they were already interested in the bug causing the problem.

"The CDC asked if NIH was planning to investigate every disease outbreak every time the states asked for help," said Dr. David Sencer, who joined the Public Health Service in 1955, came to the CDC in 1960 and was its director from 1966 to 1977. "They said, 'Certainly not. Only the interesting ones.' "

The new agency solved the conflict by promising to at least look into every outbreak that a state asked about. But the plan had an intrinsic flaw: Though the CDC had engineers, entomologists, and lab scientists left from its malaria work, it had relatively few epidemiologists. In other words, it had plenty of personnel to devise and apply solutions to public health problems, but it was thinly supplied with the researchers who could verify that a problem was occurring in the first place.

The problem was not the CDC's alone: Epidemiologists were in short supply across the country. The first academic department that taught the discipline in the United States was founded in 1919 at Johns Hopkins University. In the next twenty-seven years, many epidemiology graduates went directly to other universities, securing jobs in a field that was just beginning to grow. For the most part, they focused on calculations of risk factors and causes of disease rather than involving themselves in real-time outbreaks. It was a shift from the actions of the man whom the field considered its icon: John Snow, a London doctor who in 1854 mapped cases of cholera in a London neighborhood, and then shut down the outbreak by recommending that authorities take the handle off the neighborhood's water pump.

The nascent CDC wanted workers in the John Snow tradition, but it had relatively little to offer the academic epidemiologists who had already opted to do pure—and well-compensated—research. It found one: an associate professor at Hopkins, named Alexander Duncan Langmuir, who believed that epidemiologists needed as much as possible to come face-to-face with raw data in the field. In 1949, Langmuir agreed to come to the CDC as its chief epidemiologist, a post he would hold for twenty-one years.

He had little success, at first, getting others to join him. In a memoir article published in 1980, ten years after he retired, Langmuir confessed that his first nationwide recruiting campaign netted only "two young physicians who were genuinely interested but totally untrained." Faced with a dearth of qualified candidates to be CDC epidemiologists, Langmuir proposed a novel solution: The agency would grow its own. He would find young physicians who had the qualities he wanted, and train them to be epidemiologists after they were hired.

The newly conceived program received a boost from an unexpected source: the start of the Korean War.

The conflict began in June 1950. Within months, the decision to commit troops revived wartime mechanisms for training and supporting forces in the field that had been on hold since the end of World War II. The ramp-up included a military draft for physicians, scheduled to start in July 1951. However, the rules of the draft included a provision allowing doctors to opt out of military service if they agreed to spend two years in the Public Health Service instead. Physicians quickly took advantage of the loophole: In September 1950, only three months after the war began, Langmuir received the first letters from physicians asking to spend their two years of service at the CDC.

————

Epi boot camp broke down into distinct parts. Mornings held courses in methods of statistical analysis, interview techniques, and respecting the rights of patients. In the afternoons, the class reviewed accounts of past investigations, absorbing a thirdhand sense of what it felt like to land in an unfamiliar place and be handed responsibility for the health of strangers.

In the middle of the first week, Hamilton led a small group through a 1999 investigation that began with seven children hospitalized with bloody diarrhea near Albany, New York. One child had developed hemolytic uremic syndrome, a life-threatening disorder that includes loss of red blood cells and kidney failure. Lab analysis showed the child was infected with *Escherichia coli O157:H7,* a foodborne bacteria that releases a potent toxin. All seven children had attended the Washington County Fair nearby. So had more than 100,000 local residents. The New York state Department of Health had called the CDC for help.

"Is this an outbreak?" Hamilton asked.

"An outbreak is more cases than expected in a certain time and place," replied Waimar Tun, a Ph.D. epidemiologist who had worked in Bangladesh and Tibet. "We don't know what that baseline would be."

"So is it worth investigating?" Hamilton prodded.

"The health department asked us to investigate," said Angela McGowan, the attorney. "When they ask us, don't we have to go?"

Hamilton nodded. "The No. 1 reason we do outbreak investigations is to control disease," he said. "The second most important reason to do this is public concern: This is a life-threatening disease. And the third reason is, they are good training for what we do, and responding to public and political concern is an important part of what we do."

He walked them through the steps to be considered. How would they educate themselves about the organism? What supplies should they consider taking with them? If there are additional cases, how will they find them? When they draw a graph of the cases, what will it look like, and what will it tell them about the kind of outbreak it is?

At the end of the exercise, they learned that the seven children were the first indicator of an epidemic. Within a month, there were 761 known cases, and possibly 5,000 all together; sixty-five people were hospitalized, and two died. After a study of the patients and an environmental investigation, the source of the bacteria was found in a fairground well contaminated by cattle manure. It was one of the largest E. coli outbreaks in history.

Hamilton pointed out that the three EIS officers who were sent to the outbreak had no idea how widely the illness would spread, or whether they themselves were at risk.

"It is vital that you take care of yourselves," he said. "If you get sick, you will not do anyone any good."

———

Doctors' apprehensiveness about going to war had given Langmuir his first slate of epidemiologists-to-be, but it was broader fears about the Korean conflict that truly shaped the EIS. The rise of Cold War tensions had produced deep anxiety in the United States about the possible use of biological weapons, either smuggled covertly into the country or delivered by the long-distance missile systems that the Cold War arms race was rapidly producing. The start of the Korean War amplified those fears. China, which became the United States' chief opponent, had experience with biological weapons: Japan had used them against the Chinese in World War II, and had built weapons-research facilities in the part of China it occupied. (Popular anxiety about China's germ-warfare plans ignored or failed to realize that significant amounts of biological-weapons knowledge had been collected after the war not by China, but by the United States, which granted immunity in exchange for testimony to the heads of Japan's germ warfare program, Unit 731.)

Once the conflict began, the U.S. government evaluated what was known about biological weapons research and concluded that germ warfare directed against the United States was a real risk. A civil defense manual published in December 1950 stated flatly: "An enemy could employ . . . biological warfare against us effectively."

Langmuir—who as the government's chief epidemiologist was a consultant to the U.S. Army's own biological warfare program at Fort Detrick, Maryland—concurred. In a speech he gave in February 1951 in Kansas City, he outlined the possibilities: Infectious organisms could be released inside buildings. "Specially designed bombs, shells, or other types of disseminating devices discharged from enemy aircraft or from warships offshore" could cast clouds of pathogens over cities. Water supplies could be contaminated, as well as food stores.

"One's imagination is almost unlimited when one considers the wide variety of possibilities and potentialities of this form of warfare," he concluded.

Germ warfare was still a new thought in the 1950s, so Langmuir took care to underline an essential point: Biological weapons would be most valuable to an enemy if they caused full-blown epidemics rather than scattered cases of disease. Because germ warfare is covert by definition, intentionally caused outbreaks would come as a surprise. The number of victims would overload hospitals and emergency medical services. State laboratories that would handle diagnostic samples from victims would be overwhelmed by the amount of analysis required to explain an outbreak; in addition, their scientists might never have seen the organisms likely to be used in weapons. Lacking an explanation for the cases flooding their offices, physicians would treat victims with anything that looked as though it might be effective—an approach that might uncover a useful treatment, but would waste time and drugs along the way. Quarantines would be imposed by civil authorities. Mass panic would ensue.

Langmuir was envisioning attacks in which weaponized pathogens would be delivered directly to the United States. He shortly was forced to revise his views. In June 1951, American and United Nations troops in Korea began falling seriously ill.

At first, the illness looked like flu, with severe headache, high fever, loss of appetite, and pain in the back and abdomen. The first sign of something unusual happening showed in the sick soldiers' faces: They became bright red, as though the men were sunburned. Within a few days, victims began to look puffy-faced: Fluid collected around their eye sockets, and their eyes turned pink and then red as small blood vessels broke. Pinpoint hemorrhages appeared—first on the palate, then in the armpits and along the chest and neck. The patients vomited blood. Their blood pressure crashed, sending them into shock, and then their kidneys shut down.

More than three thousand troops became sick. Almost two hundred died, most of them within a week of falling ill. When they were autopsied, their kidneys were found to be engorged with blood and dead tissue. Bewildered military doctors dubbed the illness "epidemic hemorrhagic fever." Western medical literature held no record of it—but Japanese records did. Japanese soldiers occupying Manchuria more than ten years earlier had been attacked by the same disease, which they believed was carried by field mice and transmitted to humans by mites. But there was no record of the disease ever occurring in Korea. The U.S. military's reluctance to trust the Japanese, combined with widespread anxiety over biological weapons, led to a fresh set of fears: that soldiers had been infected deliberately by an enemy.

Frightening though the cases were, they remained confined to the battlefield. But the outbreak caused Langmuir to contemplate a second possibility: that combatants in Korea might infect U.S. troops with slower-acting organisms that would not made them sick until they returned home. He imagined companies of soldiers unknowingly made to act as human weapons against their own side, a much more efficient delivery method than the bombs and shells he had described months earlier.

Langmuir's predictions appalled Mountin and the new CDC's leadership. They transformed the dearth of epidemiologists from a problem into an emergency. In a tense meeting, Mountin said: "What we need is an epidemic intelligence service."

Years later, Langmuir wrote with satisfaction: "That is what he got." The first EIS class—twenty-one physicians and an environmental engineer who had worked on malaria—reported for two years of duty in July 1951.

Three months later, Langmuir appeared in San Francisco at the annual meeting of the American Public Health Association, before an audience of staff from state and local health departments from across the country. In a speech that made the EIS concept public for the first time—partly to stimulate recruiting for the next year's class—Langmuir described why the new corps was so necessary.

"Any plan of defense against biological warfare sabotage requires trained epidemiologists, alert to all possibilities and available for call at a moment's notice anywhere in the country," he said. "To achieve the desired mobility, the activities of these epidemiologists should be coordinated by a logical federal agency. They must be immediately available, however, to any state or local health department in need."

In one paragraph, Langmuir raised the possibility of biological attack, proposed a corps of detectives to combat it, sold it as a new addition to the taxpayer-funded CDC, and most important, dangled before the overworked health department employees the promise of highly trained, unpaid help whenever they needed it. Neither Langmuir nor his audience needed to voice the next thought: Biological attacks would at first be indistinguishable from naturally occurring epidemics. The new disease detectives were intended to uncover intentionally caused outbreaks, but they were likely to help health authorities solve many other epidemics along the way.

The states needed the help. Infectious disease outbreaks were common, in part because controls were few: Penicillin had just come into wide use, and childhood immunization programs had yet to make much of an impact. Since full-time investigation of disease outbreaks would be a new undertaking, Langmuir chose his troops carefully. He looked for a specific personality type.

"I remember he would say he wanted three characteristics in his EIS officers," said J. Lyle Conrad, a physician who came to the CDC as an EIS officer in 1965 and afterward ran a division of the CDC for eleven years. "He wanted the brightest people he could get his hands on. He wanted them to be aggressive; he even wanted them to be abrasive to a degree, to make some headway against the dead wood in public health. And he wanted them to be enthusiastic. He wanted people who, if he said, All right, young man, you've been doing cancer epidemiology too long; I've got a measles outbreak in South Dakota, and you leave tomorrow, would pack his bags, leave tomorrow and land in the snow in South Dakota without batting an eye."

The CDC's willingness to dispatch an EIS officer at any hour became the hallmark of the program. "State health officials were astounded to find bright, young, responsive epidemiologists in their offices the next morning, or even sometimes the same day that they called," Langmuir wrote in 1980. "Any situation to which the term 'epidemic' could be even remotely applied was accepted as within our jurisdiction, at least for a preliminary investigation."

Langmuir's plan contained substantial risk: He effectively staked the reputation of the nascent CDC on the performance of the newly minted researchers it sent out into the field. For the agency to succeed as Mountin envisioned, it needed to be closely tied to state health departments. Those departments would not have cared how good a CDC representative's medical credentials were. The only thing that mattered to them was whether novice epidemiologists arriving from the CDC could solve the outbreaks the states were grappling with.

Out of luck or good planning—or perhaps because Langmuir was a good judge of character—the plan succeeded. The freshly trained epidemiologists who were sent out from Atlanta puzzled out the epidemics they were presented with, even if they sometimes needed to read up on the suspected problem while they were en route to the outbreak. The group quickly began to pride itself on what it called "shoe-leather epidemiology," its core technique: trekking through the landscape of an investigation, door-to-door if need be, to conduct the face-to-face interviews that would supply the data its analyses needed. It adopted a symbol that hinted at the labor involved: the outline of the sole of a shoe with a hole worn through the ball of the foot, superimposed on a globe.

Langmuir had sold the EIS to the public health establishment as an always-available source of assistance. At home at the CDC, he hit different notes. The ultimate purpose of the EIS was to make epidemiologists, in the hopes that some at least would stick with the specialty once their two years of CDC service had ended. Investigating outbreaks was one facet of training, but not the only one. The new EIS members were taught to conduct routine surveillance for undetected health problems and to sift through collections of data for unrecognized opportunities to prevent and control diseases. They were expected to write papers and to deliver presentations at scientific conferences.

In the early years, they did all of it under Langmuir's direct supervision.

"Alex was a bit of a tyrant," Sencer said. "He was very demanding. Anybody who wrote a paper had to sit down with Alex, and Alex would go through it and tell you what needed work. You'd come back two or three times, but when that paper was done, it was good."

Langmuir retired from the CDC in 1970. He died in 1993 after a second career teaching public health. The program outlived him. Between 1951 and 2002, more than 2,700 people joined the EIS. Afterward, one-third of them stayed with the CDC; another third took jobs in state health departments and other federal agencies, and one-fifth joined university faculties. Three of them became directors of the CDC; ten ended up as deans of schools of public health. Two became U.S. surgeons general. Langmuir's initial goal—creating a cadre of trained epidemiologists to spread through U.S. public health—had been achieved.

His second goal—establishing an early-warning system against domestic biological attack—gradually came to seem less relevant as the Cold War ended and the Soviet Union dismantled itself. In the world of defense intelligence, deep concern about biological weapons never abated. U.S. research into them continued, first offensive, and then defensive after germ warfare was outlawed by international treaty in 1972.

Little of that continuing disquiet, though, touched the CDC. At its Atlanta headquarters, the onetime mosquito-control bureau built itself over fifty years into the world's premier public health agency. Its mandate expanded, taking in chronic diseases, environmental health, sexually transmitted diseases, birth defects, and the acquisition and processing of millions of data-points of health statistics. It fielded teams of field and laboratory scientists who worked in dozens of countries, eradicating smallpox and curbing measles, polio, and tuberculosis. Its name became so well recognized that the People's Republic of China dubbed its own health agency the "China CDC" in tribute, though the initials are meaningless in Chinese.

Physically and psychologically, the CDC remained remote from the rest of the government, even when concerns about biological-weapon defense were renewed in the 1990s. That changed abruptly with the October 2001 revelation that an unknown assailant had launched anthrax-laden letters against media and politicians in Florida, Washington, D.C., and New York. Five people died; seventeen others were made ill. The assumption that the American homeland was safe from biological attack was permanently shattered.

The CDC realized that Langmuir's intentions for the EIS still had relevance. For the first time since the corps' founding, new members would have to be taught to counter outbreaks of disease that had been deliberately caused.

————

"I really hope," said Colonel Ted Cieslak, "that this week is a waste of all your time."

Cieslak, an Army physician, stood at the front of a windowless white classroom in a decommissioned Army hospital in Anniston, Alabama. Cieslak was chief of pediatrics at a military medical center in San Antonio, Texas, and the brother of an EIS officer from the class of 1992. The CDC had asked him to speak based on the job he used to have: He was a former division chief from the U.S. Army Medical Research Institute of Infectious Diseases, the government installation at Fort Detrick, Maryland, that had conducted all of the Pentagon's biological-weapons research.

"Until recently, biological warfare was a paragraph tucked into the back of our chemical weapons manual," he said. "But in this day and age, you are going to have to go about your business with the possibility always tucked into the back of your minds."

The members of the EIS class shifted in their seats. The CDC had bused them all to Anniston, ninety-five miles from Atlanta, thinking that the change in routine would break up the monotony of training and give the group one last chance to get to know each other. "We want them to be bonded as a group," Hamilton said. "The friendships that are made in these two years are really enduring. And if we face a situation again like the anthrax attacks, the cohesion they have developed will help to pull them through."

The class looked exhausted. After weeks of intensive schooling in recognizing natural outbreaks of disease, their brains were almost numb. They had little stamina left for five more twelve-hour days of training—even training that promised, in theory at least, to save not just the general public's lives but their own. And the bland setting—a cinder-block room inside a nondescript brick building on an overgrown military reservation—bled the reality out of what would otherwise be a course in varieties of nightmare.

However, the setting was less benign than it looked. The reservation, Fort McClellan, was the former home of the U.S. Army's school for chemical warfare. Buried on the grounds, along with German and Italian prisoners of war who died while being held there, and bomb-sniffing military dogs that had been decorated for exemplary service, were 2,200 heavily guarded tons of nerve gas, mustard gas, and Sarin. The chemical weapons were scheduled for mass incineration, but their destruction had been postponed multiple times while the Army struggled with the risks of cracking open the stockpile. Without knowing it, the EIS officers were surrounded by some of the weapons they were being trained to defend against.

Cieslak took them briskly through the basics. Category A agents, the most dangerous not only for their infectiousness, but for the panic they would inspire: anthrax, botulism, smallpox, plague, and viral hemorrhagic fevers including Ebola. Category B agents, ones that would cause more sickness though less death, such as the livestock diseases brucellosis and Q fever, and ricin, a toxin expressed from castor beans. Category C agents, newly recognized diseases that the CDC feared could be engineered into weapons, like hantavirus, which had emerged unexpectedly in the Southwest a decade earlier, and Nipah virus, which had killed one hundred people in Malaysia in 1999.

PowerPoint images clicked by with the lecture. An electron-micrograph of a virus. An image of a first responder at an anthrax hoax, hidden from head to toe behind hooded coveralls and scuba-style breathing gear. A child with full-blown smallpox infection. That drew gasps. Smallpox had been eradicated before most of the class members reached high school. None of the physicians in the group had studied it in medical school. Few people, other than intelligence analysts, had expected to have to encounter it again. But on the list of organisms likely to be deployed by a terrorist, smallpox now ranked close to the top. Because most vaccinations had ceased thirty years ago, much of the world was considered vulnerable to it. Its release could potentially cause mass outbreaks, and a faster-moving epidemic of fear.

"You should be asking yourself: What is the average terrorist thinking?" Cieslak said. "If they are seeking a strategic goal—the destruction of the United States, for instance—there are probably only four or five biological agents they are going to use. But if the terrorist's goal is not so grandiose, the list of potential agents is much longer. For the big four—anthrax, smallpox, botulism, and plague—diagnosis may actually be quite easy. Unfortunately, if it's one of the rest, your problems immediately increase."

An attack would come as a surprise, the physician reminded them. The first signs that it had happened would be the cases of illness that it caused.

"If you suspect you've been hit with a biological weapon, the rest is relatively easy," he said. "You'll be able to do the right thing, if you suspect it in time. The problem in biological defense is recognizing the attack in the first place."

Cieslak sat down. A radiation physicist, a small, dry man in a suit, took his place. He looked out at the class. Shaken out of their exhaustion, all eighty-nine of them stared back.

"Is there anyone here," he said, "who knows how to operate a Geiger counter?"

————

The EIS class members stood in a rough circle inside another Anniston classroom, two buildings away from where they had started the week. At their feet, each of them had a large plastic trash bag. The bags were twisted shut; blank name-tags with wire tails held them closed.

The bags held the essentials of the last phase of their training. They had spent most of the week listening to the possible forms a terrorist attack could take. Now, they were going to enact one. The simulation, they had been told in advance, would be a poison-gas attack. They would suit up, set up their emergency response, find and treat the victims, and then learn how to retreat without becoming victims themselves, all within the confines of the building. The simulation was expected to be stressful. Outside the building, several paramedics were standing by.

The class split up into smaller groups, trailing after instructors into separate corridors of the building. One went with Danny Garrick, a tall, broad-shouldered man with hair so short and a manner so curt he could have passed for a drill instructor. Coached by Garrick, the group opened up their bags and got acquainted with the contents: Surgical gloves, with thick electricians' gauntlets to cover them. Heavy rubber boots with clear plastic liners to make them easier to pull on. A zipped white coverall with booties, a hood, and elastic at the waist, neck, and sleeves.

"This is Tyvek," Garrick said, holding it up. "It's a good protection against particulate matter. It offers limited splash protection. If you're somewhere where it's wet, don't kneel when you're wearing this; whatever the liquid is, it will soak right through."

The last item in the bags was an air-purifying respirator: a thick clear-plastic mask mounted on a pair of filter cartridges, surrounded by a heavy rubber gasket and held on the head with wide elastic straps. The masks were a struggle to don quickly: The elastic pulled hair out of place and the gaskets sat uncomfortably on beards.

"Take deep, slow breaths," Garrick warned them. He strolled around the group, stopping at a woman who had pushed the gasket down over her bangs. He bent slowly, bringing his face level with the front of her mask, and peered in.

"That hair inside your mask is breaking the seal that's protecting you," he said, gently. "You realize, if this were a real emergency, you'd be dead right now."

The group shuffled rapidly into the training area, confronting the body on the gurney and a set of incongruous props: a stack of trash bags, a garden sprayer, and a child's plastic wading pool.

The pool and the sprayer, Garrick said, were for victims who could walk into decontamination. If nothing like them was available, trash cans would do, or buckets or a garden hose—anything that would let them rinse victims down rapidly with water, plus bleach if they could get it or soap if they could not.

"Think about the complexities here," he said. "Time is of the essence. You're going to have to move these people to medical care. If you have a parent with a child, you're going to have to decontaminate them together. If you have a blind person with a dog, you're going to have to decontaminate the dog."

Victims got washed down once with their clothes on, then again naked. They could take their clothes off themselves if they were able to, but things would go faster if the EIS cut them off instead. The trash bags served two functions: They were evidence bags for the clothing, because a terrorist attack would be considered a crime scene; and they were a modest emergency covering once the clothing was taken away.

"If you're at a hospital, you might be able to find sheets, or a stash of scrubs. If you can't then trash bags are your best substitute," Garrick said. "If you're grabbing them in a hurry, try to make sure you pick the dark ones—not the ones that are clear."

The last part of the exercise was learning how to take the suits off safely. The class members stepped into the trash bags the suits had arrived in, holding them open with their knees. The gear came off in a careful sequence: First, drop the gauntlets into the bag, peel the suit away to the knees, and step out of the boots and suit. Then, take a deep breath and hold it; pull off the respirator and gloves; tilt your face away; drop them into the bag and twist it shut; and breathe again. The last step was to label the bag with the name-tag, in case the contaminated gear was considered evidence as well.

The class members reassembled in the classroom, breathing deeply and rubbing the red marks the gaskets had left on their faces. The exercise had lasted fifty minutes. If it ever occurred in real life, it would be hours, Messanier warned them on the way out.

"If something happens, you are on your own," he said. "You will be on your own for at least eight to twelve hours. That's the minimum amount of time it will take for the rest of the feds to show up."

TWO

Polio

1955, Atlanta

APRIL 12, 1955 WAS AN EXTRAORDINARY DAY in America. Church bells rang, though it was a Tuesday. Cars honked their horns nonstop, and factories and firehouses rang their sirens. Shoppers rushed into stores to listen to their radios. Women, and some men, wept in the streets.

The news that galvanized the nation was not the start of a war, or the end of one. It was the announcement in Ann Arbor, Michigan, of the development of a vaccine against polio.

The achievement was electric because the disease itself was so frightening. Polio, known for thousands of years, had attacked the United States with extraordinary force since about the turn of the century. Every summer, it seemed, epidemics ripped through small towns and at least one major city: There had been 27,000 cases just in New York in 1916, and close to 58,000 nationwide in 1952, the worst year on record. Polio was loathed and feared not just because it was relentless, but because it was selective. Overwhelmingly, it attacked children, turning robust toddlers and teenagers into limp, feverish cripples almost overnight. The disease was cruelly random—one child in a family could be stricken while siblings remained unaffected—and its paralysis was irreversible. The higher up the body the paralysis occurred, the more desperate the case became, until doctors were forced to encase victims in the primitive respirators known as "iron lungs."

Polio was an agent of social disruption. If a child developed it, health authorities would lock the family into quarantine; more than one case in a neighborhood could trigger the closing of theaters, playgrounds, swimming pools, and schools. Families with means sent their children into exile to avoid it, packing them off to summer homes or to Europe with nannies and grandparents. Income and flight, though, were insufficient protection: The best known polio victim in America had been President Franklin Delano Roosevelt, son of a rich and well-connected family, who developed the disease at the age of thirty-nine on the secluded island off the coast of Maine where his family had summered for years.

The day that the vaccine was announced was the tenth anniversary of Roosevelt's death. That was no accident: The huge vaccine trial coordinated by the University of Michigan had been funded by the National Foundation for Infantile Paralysis, the "March of Dimes" run by FDR's former law partner Basil O'Connor. More than 1.8 million schoolchildren in forty-four states had participated. The results were unequivocal: The vaccine effectively prevented polio paralysis. The summer monster had been vanquished. Vaccinations began immediately nationwide.

The jubilation was short-lived. On April 25, an infant who had been vaccinated nine days earlier was carried into the emergency ward of the Michael Reese Hospital in Chicago. Both of the baby's legs were paralyzed.

————

In Atlanta, Dr. Neal Nathanson had been waiting for something to do. Nathanson was twenty-eight, a fine-boned man with large glasses who wore his hair cropped close to his skull. Until a few weeks earlier, he had been an internal medicine resident at the University of

Chicago, finishing his first year of specialization after a general internship and planning eventually to become a neurologist. Then a draft notice arrived.

Nathanson thought he had escaped military service: He was so severely nearsighted that a draft board physician had immediately classified him 4-F, unacceptable. This notice, though, was not for the general military draft for which he had already been considered and rejected; it was for the doctors' draft, a holdover from the Korean War. The doctors' draft had less stringent physical standards, and only one main requirement: A man had to have graduated from medical school. Nathanson had—from Harvard, in 1953.

And that was the source of the trouble. The notice had been sent by the draft board in Cambridge, Massachusetts, the home base of Harvard University. Relations between the mixed-income town and the powerful school had foundered periodically during most of Harvard's three-hundred-plus years of existence. The most recent flare-up expressed itself in an apparent decision by Cambridge's draft board to cause maximum difficulty for anyone associated with Harvard, including its newly minted doctors, who actually studied on a campus across the Charles River in Boston. In most areas, draft notices arrived during the winter, summoning new physicians to induction as military officers the following July 1. Nathanson's notice called for him to report for duty in thirty days, with the rank of private first class.

The irony, though the draft board never realized it, was that they were persecuting one of their own. Nathanson had graduated from both Harvard College and Harvard Medical School; the board knew that, because they had his medical school address. What they did not know was that he was a townie, born and bred on the Cambridge side of the river. He had no particular desire to be a military physician, and no interest in starting as a buck private. Being treated like one of Cambridge's rich intruders made him even less inclined to cooperate.

Uncertain what to do next, he turned for advice to the Chicago medical school's chief resident, a man named J. Thomas Grayston. Grayston had studied at University of Chicago since 1947—he had bachelor's, master's, and medical degrees from its various divisions—

but his education was interrupted for two of those years: He had been part of the first Epidemic Intelligence Service class in 1951.

Alexander Langmuir, the EIS's leader and the government's chief epidemiologist, was the only powerful person Grayston knew. He placed a call. By coincidence, Langmuir was short an officer; one of the physicians selected for the EIS the previous summer had decided to take another job. He offered the slot to Nathanson. On April 1, Nathanson enrolled in the EIS class of 1955, three months early and without taking the mandatory summer training course.

He could have used the training. He had had even less exposure to disease detection than most new doctors: His medical school class had feuded with their epidemiology professor and refused to attend most of the class sessions. Unsure what he was getting into, he moved to Atlanta and settled into an office down the hall from Langmuir, in the small downtown building that housed the nine-year-old CDC. Most of the EIS class had been sent out to state posts to work. Left to himself, Nathanson got acquainted with the agency and wondered what his first assignment would be like.

In the last week of April, Langmuir poked his head around the door, asked after Nathanson's health, and made him the chief of the brand-new polio surveillance unit—a grand-sounding group that consisted of Nathanson, a statistician EIS officer named William Jackson Hall, and a secretary.

It was three days after the infant had been carried into the Chicago hospital, and the polio vaccination program was already beginning to fall apart. Nine more cases of paralysis had been found, in California, Georgia, and Idaho; one of the Idaho cases, the father of a vaccinated child, had died. Los Angeles, Oakland, and Albany had cancelled their vaccination programs; Philadelphia suspended its inoculations and then, in confusion, restarted them. All ten cases were linked to vaccine made by one manufacturer, Cutter Laboratories of Berkeley, California. Surgeon General Leonard Scheele had ordered the Cutter vaccine, one of six being used in the campaign, yanked from the market. Simultaneously, he had pulled Langmuir and the CDC into tracking down what had gone wrong.

In an interview he gave to *The New York Times,* Scheele described what the CDC would be seeking, in the process making the mission of the EIS broadly public for the first time. "It will be 'epidemic intelligence,'" he said, "in the sense of intelligence in battle."

On the day he gave the interview, 4 million doses of vaccine had already been administered.

——————

The polio vaccination program had been a gamble from the start—both whether it would work, and whether the public would accept it. Polio vaccines had a poor history: Two earlier attempts in 1935, headed by scientists Maurice Brodie and John Kolmer, had failed. The Brodie vaccine trial vaccinated 9,000 children and adults; three became paralyzed, and one died. The Kolmer vaccine was used on 11,000 subjects; nine children and an adult developed paralysis, and five of the children died. Investigators thought at the time that the Brodie cases were natural polio, occurring because the vaccine did not protect its recipients. The Kolmer cases were much more troubling: They were caused by the vaccine itself.

The failures were a setback for the National Foundation, which had funded the Brodie trial. The organization had been paying for polio research since 1934, three years before it was officially incorporated; it had started as a group of FDR intimates who raised money for Warm Springs, Georgia, a polio-treatment property that Roosevelt bought after he became disabled. The foundation paid for the treatment and rehabilitation of any polio victim in the United States who needed financial help. It also ran programs to train doctors and nurses in surgical and physical-therapy treatments. From its beginnings, though, the group's ultimate goal had been preventing cases of polio from occurring. A vaccine seemed the only plausible path.

In 1951, O'Connor had met researchers John Enders and Jonas Salk aboard an ocean liner in mid-Atlantic. All three were returning from a European polio meeting, where Enders, a Harvard bacteriologist, had been feted for developing a method of growing poliovirus in tissue cultures, an achievement for which he and two colleagues would win a Nobel Prize in 1954. Before the Harvard team's discovery, scientific work with polio had been confined to infecting animals and trying to extract virus from their tissues after they were killed. Enders's breakthrough allowed researchers to grow large amounts of pure virus, giving them the raw material for vaccine research. Salk, who was only thirty-seven, had made use of Enders's discovery: He had grown quantities of poliovirus in his University of Pittsburgh lab, and then developed a vaccine based on virus that was killed by mixing it with formalin, a lab preservative. Salk had helped develop the first influenza vaccine, which used killed virus; he believed that using a killed poliovirus would induce immunity to that disease as well.

Given the unhappy history of the Brodie and Kolmer attempts, Salk's killed-virus vaccine had obvious appeal. A killed virus, by definition, could not cause an infection; if it did not cause infection, it could not lead to unintended cases of paralysis. The work intrigued O'Connor, who brought Salk into the circle of polio researchers backed by the foundation. With the group's huge resources behind him, Salk tested his vaccine on small groups: first the mentally disabled residents of a state school, then children who were recent victims of polio who lived in a private orphanage, and finally child and adult volunteers in public schools near Pittsburgh. In 1953, he published his results and came to O'Connor with a proposition: The vaccine was good enough to test broadly. A statistically significant trial would need thousands of participants, and cost $7 million.

The foundation agreed to support Salk, and the yearlong trial began in April 1954. It was actually two trials: In one, second graders in certain areas were vaccinated, but first and third graders were not; they were merely watched for their rate of naturally occurring polio. The foundation's advisors worried that the design might not be statistically solid, so they added a second arm to the study: In it, both first and second graders were given either the vaccine or a placebo, an inert injection that looked and felt identical to the actual vaccine. Over both branches of the study, 441,000 children were given the vaccine, with another 201,000 receiving placebos and almost 1.2 million observed as a gauge of infection rates.

The vaccinations took three months, but tabulating the data sent in by thousands of volunteers took another nine. The tabulation was performed by an office that was completely separate from Salk and his lab and was set up to handle the trial's millions of pieces of information. It was called the Poliomyelitis Vaccine Evaluation Center, based in Ann Arbor and run by Dr. Thomas Francis Jr., who had supervised Salk's flu research. Francis held the results close until the last minute. The foundation, though, suspected that the trial would go well enough—fear of polio was so great that people would demand Salk's vaccine even if it only worked a little—and so they began looking beyond the day when the results would be announced. Led by O'Connor, the foundation negotiated with drug manufacturers to make several million batches of the Salk vaccine while the trial was going on, enough to begin a limited nationwide campaign as soon as the trial report was delivered and federal licensing authorities could be persuaded to sign off. Six companies agreed to take the $9 million order: Parke-Davis and Co. and Eli Lilly and Co., who had supplied the vaccines for the trial; and Cutter, Pitman-Moore Co., Sharp & Dohme, and Wyeth Laboratories.

O'Connor's gamble was rewarded. On April 12, Francis delivered the eagerly awaited report in a University of Michigan auditorium; outside, reporters climbed over each other to grab copies and race to the phones. Among the inoculated children, Francis said, there had been 119 cases of polio; among the placebo group, less than half as large, there had been 142 cases. The vaccine worked—though it was not perfect. It was 60 percent effective against type 1 poliovirus, the most frequent cause of polio in the United States, and 90 percent effective against the less common types 2 and 3. Among the masses of data gathered by the volunteers, there was no record of any adverse reactions. Oveta Culp Hobby, secretary of Health, Education and Welfare, signed the licensing papers before the end of the afternoon. Distribution began immediately.

So did vaccination. Of the first Cutter cases, one had been vaccinated on April 14, one on April 15, and the other four on April 16.

———

The CDC faced two essential questions: Were the paralysis cases naturally occurring polio that the vaccine had failed to prevent? Or, despite the killed-virus guarantee, were they caused by the vaccine itself?

There was no way to answer them without knowing more about the cases. That meant finding them, to start with. The unofficial count, reported by newspapers, was growing rapidly: By April 29, there were twenty-six, in six states. The next day, there were thirty-five. One week later, there were forty-four. The unofficial counts were insufficient, though: Nathanson and Hall needed to know about every apparent case of polio in the country. Whether they were naturally occurring, vaccine-associated, or misidentified would emerge once the true size of the problem was defined.

With Langmuir looking over their shoulders, the two EIS members sketched out the questions that they needed state health officials to answer for every case of polio that could be linked to a vaccination. That took in more than just the five- to nine-year-olds who were supposed to be the first to be vaccinated. Most of the first lots of vaccine had been given to health departments, but some had gone to private physicians; some of them, wanting to please their patients, had vaccinated infants and adults as well. And because the first set of cases included a man who had not gotten the shot—but who might have caught polio from a child who did get the vaccine—the investigators realized they needed to ask about family and neighborhood cases as well.

Scheele had ordered every state to name one person to collect data for the CDC. On April 29, Nathanson and Hall phoned and telegraphed the first version of their questionnaire to their state counterparts, including twenty-four EIS members who were already working out in the field. It was an exhaustive list. At a minimum, they wanted the victims' initials, address, age and gender, onset of symptoms, onset and site of paralysis, and date of vaccination. After that, they asked for detailed symptoms, lab analysis of a spinal tap and stool specimens, evaluations of muscle strength by a physical therapist, the location where the vaccination had taken place, the vaccination status and illnesses of every friend or family member who came in contact with the victim, and the names and addresses of the treating physician and the local investigator.

Two days later, on May 1, the team published their first Poliomyelitis Surveillance Report. They did it again the next day, and for thirty-five days in a row, and then once a week for many weeks thereafter.

"None of the reports we got back were complete," Nathanson said. "I don't remember one. So you would be on the phone for each case, for every detail of each case, and every detail came from someone different whom you had to call. There was duplication. There were questionable cases, and there were cases that were clearly not polio. And we were doing this for the entire country, day after day."

The researchers had also been ordered to interrogate every health department about the vaccine that had come into their area: which manufacturer had supplied the vaccine, how many doses had arrived, who had gotten hold of them, and how many had been administered. Those were crucial details for deciphering whether any other manufacturer's vaccine was causing problems. If only one company's vaccine could be implicated in the polio cases, the problem might lie with that manufacturer. But if several companies were at fault, the problem might lie not with their procedures, but with the vaccine recipe. If that were the case, the entire vaccination program might have to be cancelled—and the twenty-year search for a polio vaccine might have to begin anew.

The six manufacturers' vaccines had not been distributed evenly across the country; with the release happening so rapidly, each company's product ended up close to where it was manufactured. Because Cutter was a California company, the largest proportion of its vaccine had stayed in the West, in California, Arizona, Nevada, New Mexico, Idaho, and Hawaii. Small amounts, though, had been sent east as well. By the time it was pulled from the market on April 27, almost 400,000 doses had been administered in twenty-six states.

In most of the country, vaccinations were continuing, though anxiety over them was rising. Finding what doses went where, and whether they were associated with cases, was painstaking, grueling work.

"We worked from seven in the morning til nine at night," Nathanson said. "We'd go home and drop, and start again the next morning. It was like being in an emergency room, at the height of a crisis, all the time."

Outside Atlanta, the urgency mounted. On April 28, the surgeon general dispatched two National Institutes of Health researchers to scour the Cutter plant for any sign of problems. On April 30, the Laboratory of Biologics Control—the predecessor to the Food and Drug Administration—told vaccine manufacturers to suspend making any more vaccine until the situation was clarified. On May 5, an emergency research summit at NIH recommended that teams of scientists be sent to inspect every vaccine-manufacturing plant.

On May 7, the count of paralysis cases rose to fifty. Two of them had received a vaccine that was not made by Cutter. The government halted the entire vaccination program.

———

Most of the Cutter vaccine had supplied the vaccination programs in California, the company's home state, and Idaho. To the beleaguered investigators, that was a piece of good news.

Polio is a warm-weather disease. Mid-April in Idaho was not warm; the local polio season had not started. The coincidence gave the researchers a natural laboratory in which they could examine the outbreak's central issue: Were the new cases of paralysis a striking coincidence, or were they incontrovertibly associated with the vaccine?

Idaho gave them an answer. In the previous five years, according to state records, there had been about one case of polio per week between the middle of April and the end of June. In any one of those years, during that time period, there had been no more than eleven cases. In 1955, there were eighty-eight. The difference was far too large to be labeled coincidence.

The data that Nathanson and Hall were wrestling out of the states backed up their Idaho observation. In the mountains of reports pouring into the CDC, trends began to emerge. In every community, cases of paralysis tended to occur in waves; that suggested that each cluster had a cause—a single source—rather than occurring randomly. Moreover, the waves resembled each other; in each instance, cases occurred among the vaccinated within four to fifteen days of vaccination, and among their contacts within eight to thirty days. That implied that each case experienced an incubation period of the same length—and that the second-generation family cases became sick within the span of two incubation periods, their child's plus their own.

To double-check their findings, the researchers mapped the number of paralysis cases across the country against the weeks in which they had occurred. They did the same for previous years, and then compared the trend lines. The difference was dramatic. From 1951 through 1954, polio cases started in late spring and zoomed steadily upward past the end of July. The 1955 line had two peaks in early summer and fell almost to zero by the last week of July. Those two peaks were the first and third weeks of May—exactly one and two incubation periods after the Cutter vaccine was pulled from the market.

There remained the question of whether Cutter was the only company at fault. Other manufacturers were accused of causing paralysis cases: By May 14, among just the vaccinated schoolchildren, one case was blamed on Parke-Davis, four on Pitman, seven on Wyeth, and twenty-eight on Lilly, which had supplied more vaccine than all the other manufacturers put together. Forty-one cases had been laid at Cutter's door.

No one pretended that the vaccine was 100 percent effective; though none of the authorities stressed the point amidst the celebration, some cases of polio had been expected all along. The researchers devised an equation that took in numbers of vaccinated children, school populations in the affected states and local polio trends in recent years. They called the result an "expected-observed comparison" and used it to evaluate the cases linked to each manufacturer. The findings backed up what they had already discovered. The other manufacturers' cases of polio were within predictable limits; Cutter's cases were five times higher than they should have been. The gap between the Cutter cases and those of the other manufacturers was so significant that it suggested one conclusion: There was something wrong with the Cutter vaccine.

"Indicting Cutter was relatively easy," Nathanson said. "But it was like the difference between identifying a perpetrator and having a case that you can bring to court. We needed the documentation."

To solidify their case, the researchers turned the same technique on the Cutter vaccine by itself, comparing the number of cases with the expected rate of polio in areas where that vaccine had been administered. Their finding surprised them. Cutter had released eight manufacturing runs—what it called "production pools"—of vaccine. The rate of paralysis cases, it turned out, was not the same across all production pools. Six of the pools, used for 268,900 vaccinations, produced 41 cases of paralysis. Two of them, used for 121,700 shots, produced 149 cases.

To make the comparisons even, the researchers used the simple statistical technique of turning the raw numbers into ratios with a common denominator of 100,000. That threw a spotlight on the difference between the pools. For every 100,000 people vaccinated, six of the pools had caused 15 cases of paralysis, and two of them had caused 122. Nathanson and Hall appeared to have their culprit: Two lots of vaccine, representing a tiny fraction of the more than 6 million that had been used.

One more piece of evidence clinched their case. They went back to the Idaho data and looked more closely at the details of the paralysis cases. They noticed something unusual. In most of the patients, the paralysis started close to where they had been vaccinated—which was occasionally in the thigh or buttock, for babies, but most commonly in the upper arm. The paralysis always occurred in the same arm where the shot had been given.

That made no sense. The progression of polio was well documented; overwhelmingly, it started in the legs and then ascended through the body. A case of polio that began in an arm and moved down the spine was unnatural. But it was also familiar: The same pattern had been noticed after the Kolmer vaccinations in 1935—the vaccinations that had been determined, after careful study, to have caused nine cases of polio paralysis.

A final pass through the data confirmed the association. One particular group of patients was most likely to have paralysis that began in the inoculated limb. It was the same group of patients whose shots had come from the two implicated production pools.

The CDC had an answer, and the outbreak had a culprit. The research satisfied Scheele, the surgeon general. On May 24, he announced the official relaunch of the vaccination program, allowing use of vaccine made by the manufacturers who had been inspected and approved by the Public Health Service investigators over the past three weeks. Scheele held back from the market only the two implicated lots of Cutter vaccine.

"The epidemiologic data," he said, "present strong presumptive evidence of a cause and effect relationship between the cases of paralytic poliomyelitis and the use of two lots of Cutter vaccine."

———

The effect was known, but the cause still was not—until June 5. In a press conference that day, Scheele announced the results of the Cutter plant inspection. Live poliovirus had been found in samples of the Cutter vaccine.

The answer to the question of who was at fault—the vaccine maker, or the vaccine recipe—turned out to be both. There was an unanticipated flaw in the Salk process. The formalin that was used to kill the virus rendered it inert by coagulating the proteins on its surface, making it impossible for the virus to attach to cells. When the proteins coagulated, though, they turned sticky, allowing adjacent viruses in the vaccine solution to clump together. Every so often, in the center of an aggregated clump, a poliovirus particle would survive unharmed.

The clumping problem was an inherent risk in the basic chemistry of Salk's research, but it was exacerbated by the scale of mass vaccine production. It was a visible problem, investigators testified afterward: At the bottom of the giant glass carboys used to make vaccine, you could sometimes see a fine sediment resting. Those were the aggregates, falling out of the solution and sometimes harboring an infectious virus inside. All of the manufacturers had filtered their vaccine products at some point in the manufacturing process, to fine out the sediment. At Cutter, some of the live virus had slipped through.

The final toll of the Cutter incident was 260 cases of polio: 94 among those who were vaccinated, 126 among their family members, and 40 among friends and members of their communities. Ten of the recipients died.

The vaccination program was not destroyed, but it was dented. Despite the surgeon general's all-clear in late May, most local vaccination campaigns did not resume until autumn. The delay was due in part to additional government regulation on vaccine manufacturing: Manufacturers were required to make filtration the final step in manufacturing, and were not allowed to release any vaccine to market until five successive manufacturing runs tested pure. But the delay was due as well to profound public distrust. Fear of polio never abated, but enthusiasm for the vaccine was blunted for some months. It revived, though: By 1961, U.S. children received more than 400 million doses of polio vaccine—without a single case of vaccine-associated polio.

It took almost a month for the Cutter polio problem to be solved. The answers seemed to come rapidly—but for the investigators, the search had lasted almost too long. Nathanson, who went on to a distinguished career as a research virologist and is now professor emeritus of microbiology at the University of Pennsylvania, has never shaken the sense that the Cutter crisis was controlled barely in time.

"If the program had been closed down for longer—or the basic vaccine formula had been proved to be unsafe—this could have had ripple effects that would have lasted for years," Nathanson said. "It could have led to a disenchantment with all vaccines. It would have been a public health disaster."

THREE

West Nile Virus
August–October 2002,
Atlanta

LATE IN THE DAY ON JULY 30, 2002, a teenage girl who lived near Atlanta was severely injured in a car accident. She was taken to a local emergency department, where the staff fought to save her. Nothing they did, though, could arrest the massive bleeding caused by her injuries. On July 31, she was declared brain-dead.

By the next evening, the young woman's kidneys, heart, and liver had been harvested, and within twenty-four hours they were transplanted into four chronically ill people. One kidney went to a thirty-one-year-old Georgia woman and the other to a thirty-eight-year-old Georgia man; both of them had severe high blood pressure that had destroyed their own kidneys. The young woman's heart was transplanted into the chest of a sixty-three-year-old man in Florida with congestive heart failure. Her liver went to a seventy-one-year-old Florida woman who had suffered a double attack by liver cancer and hepatitis C.

All four operations went smoothly. The younger patients, who were both treated at Emory University Hospital in Atlanta, recovered quickly. The thirty-one-year-old woman went home on August 6, and the thirty-eight-year-old man left the hospital one day later.

For more than a week, they did fine. On August 13, the thirty-one-year-old woman developed a rash on her chest and neck; three days later, she began to run a fever. On August 18, after a day of backache and diarrhea, she was taken back to Emory. The next day, the thirty-eight-year-old man who had gotten the other kidney also developed a moderate fever, along with a severe headache, diarrhea, and muscle aches. The next day, he went back to the hospital too.

To the mystification of their doctors, both of them got rapidly worse. Fever after an operation suggested an infection; the immune-suppressing drugs that transplant recipients take to prevent rejection would make it easy for an infection to take hold. Courses of antibiotics, though, did nothing to improve the patients' condition. Both had trouble speaking, became confused, and lapsed into unconsciousness. On August 22, the woman was put on a ventilator; on August 23, doctors did the same for the man.

The next thing the Emory doctors did was to call the surgeons who had operated on the two Florida patients. They did not like what they found. The man who received the heart had never left the hospital where his transplant took place, Jackson Memorial Hospital in Miami. He had spiked a fever August 12, lost control of the muscles in his legs, and then fallen into a coma. He had been put on a ventilator on August 21. The woman with the liver had fared slightly better: She had just been discharged that day from the Jacksonville branch of the Mayo Clinic, 350 miles from Miami. But she had had weakness and diarrhea, and fever that resisted treatment, for two weeks.

Unexplained fever and altered mental status in two patients treated in the same hospital would have been bad enough. Unexplained fever and other identical symptoms in four patients in three cities—four patients linked by a single organ donor—was much worse.

———

August 23 was a Friday. The phone call launching the investigation came into the Georgia Division of Public Health just as Martha Iwamoto was packing up for the weekend. The thirty-four-year-old pediatrician had been out of EIS training for almost three weeks.

EIS members are given a choice between working at one of the CDC's divisions, or being placed in a state health department as a CDC representative. Both options had benefits and drawbacks. Choosing Atlanta—or even the agency's subsidiary offices, in locations such as Cincinnati, Fort Collins, Colorado, and Morgantown, West Virginia—meant being close to the heart of the agency. Corps members stood in line with senior scientists in the spartan cafeteria; they ran the chance of being in the room when national health policy was being debated. But being at the CDC also meant choosing a specialty. The agency was divided into centers and institutes; infectious diseases, chronic diseases, birth defects, workplace injuries, environmental health, sexually transmitted diseases, accidental injuries, immunizations, and health statistics were the main ones. Then it was subdivided into divisions, branches, and offices. The National Center for Chronic Disease Prevention and Health Promotion, for instance, held divisions that dealt with diabetes, cancer, reproductive health, tobacco use, adolescent health, and obesity. To work in the National Center for Infectious Diseases, the CDC's largest unit, meant choosing among bacterial, viral, parasitic, and insect-borne diseases, and then opting for hepatitis over herpesvirus, or foodborne illness over strep.

Organizationally, state health departments were flatter. They were likely to have a chief, the state's health director, and a lead epidemiologist. Beyond that, there could be anywhere from a few staff members to several hundred, depending on the size of the state's population and the generosity of its legislature. To go to a state health department as an EIS officer meant sacrificing the chance to specialize, as well as the possibility of shaping policy and regulation. What it offered instead was breadth of experience: State officers were expected to grapple with infectious disease outbreaks and environmental problems and questions about childhood shots, sometimes all at once. There might be less supervision than at headquarters, and fewer experts to seek counsel from, but as compensation there was a much thinner filter between public health workers and the public.

Martha Iwamoto had liked that trade-off. A graduate of a small southern liberal arts college and the Medical College of Georgia who had done residency at the University of Virginia, she had come to the corps after two years of private practice and a year earning a public health degree. She was a small, slender woman, with thick, shoulder-length black hair and stylish, rimless eyeglasses. She was very smart and very shy, with a strong sense of privacy. Her two years as a working pediatrician, counseling parents who were unsure when to vaccinate their children, had given her a glimpse of the ways that public health policies played out in real life. Spending her EIS years in a state, she thought, would let her explore that intersection a bit more. "At a state level," she said, "you can see whether any recommendation that comes from the CDC will actually work."

As EIS assignments went, the Georgia public health division was actually a middle choice: It was incontrovertibly a state health department independent from the CDC, but it was less than five miles from CDC headquarters, and its staff was larded with former agency employees. The division was headed by Dr. Kathleen Toomey, a tall, friendly family-practice physician with a head-spinning resume: She had graduated from Smith College, gone to the Amazon Basin on a Fulbright to study native healing practices, earned medical and public health degrees at Harvard, and then spent three years north of the Arctic Circle as a Public Health Service doctor. She was reputed to have been the inspiration for the Manhattan-doctor-goes-to-Alaska TV show *Northern Exposure,* though she was second-generation Czechoslovakian from Pennsylvania coal-mining country instead of Jewish from New York. Working for her was Dr. Paul Blake, a reserved man with a close-trimmed beard and a bone-dry sense of humor who was several inches taller than his ebullient boss. He had grown up in Angola, the child of missionary parents, and come back to the States for schooling. He had a medical degree from Boston University and a public health degree from Harvard; he and Toomey had both been residents at University of Washington in Seattle, ten years apart. He had spent twenty-six years at the CDC, rising through the ranks of its enteric diseases branch, which dealt with bacteria such as salmonella that attacked through the gut. He was very well known at the CDC, and very popular. When he retired, he had come to the Georgia division; he had ended up as state epidemiologist, Toomey's second-in-command.

Toomey and Blake had both been EIS members, she in 1987 and he in 1969. Thirteen members of their staff had been in the EIS also, more than in any other state health department. Among EIS slots, the epidemiology unit at the Georgia department was one of the most desirable. It had been Martha's first choice for an assignment. That she had gotten it suggested that she had been Georgia's first choice as well.

When the CDC called back that Friday evening to confirm that the Atlanta organ donor was somehow at the center of an outbreak—four people in two states with fevers of unknown origin, three of them so sick they were unable to breathe on their own—Toomey and Blake signaled their confidence in their new EIS officer. They handed the investigation to her.

She was not on her own, though. Langmuir had designed the Epidemic Intelligence Service to mimic the medical residency he had endured at Boston City Hospital, a sprawling, underfunded inner-city campus. In fifty-one years, the CDC had not significantly changed his model. In residency, newly graduated doctors learn to be physicians by caring for patients, sticking with each case through work shifts that can last up to thirty-six hours. The new doctors always have backup, teams of more senior professionals who give them advice and sign off on their decisions, but the backup stays in the background except in emergencies: The new doctors interpret symptoms, order treatments, and are held responsible if things go badly. In the EIS, the "patient" was the outbreak; the epidemiologist-in-training led the investigation and chose the lines of inquiry, but more experienced supervisors were usually close at hand. The two experiences were not exactly parallel, though. Investigating an outbreak required a potentially jarring shift in perspective, from focusing intently on a single patient to considering many at once.

Because the four cases of fever crossed state lines, Martha had more backup than a state-based EIS officer would normally get—not just her Georgia supervisors, but CDC specialists in infections that occur inside hospitals. It gave some bench depth to an investigation forced to start with broad questions: Had the accident victim been sick in some unrecognized fashion? Had the organs been contaminated when they were removed from her body? Were the four patients—who before the transplants had all been seriously ill—simply the victims of coincidence and bad luck?

"These were patients who were immunosuppressed, who had just undergone dangerous surgery," Martha said. "It would not be unexpected for them to have a complicated course of recovery. It wasn't clear what was going on."

The task before her would be to find out everything she could about the patients: Where they had come from. How long they had been in the hospital before the transplants happened. Whether there was anything very similar, or very different, about their treatment once the transplants took place. Perhaps they had all picked up the same infection, one of the many bugs that lurked in hospital environments. All of the patients had been given multiple blood tests once their illnesses were discovered, as well as lumbar punctures to check for bacterial meningitis and viral infections. The remaining blood and cerebrospinal fluid had been saved. They were pulled from the hospital's freezers and tested again.

On August 29, the man who had received the kidney died.

His doctors prevailed on his family to allow an autopsy. They consented. It revealed that he had died of encephalitis, an overwhelming inflammation of the brain. The swelling had squeezed the base of the brain through the narrow opening at the bottom of the skull, compressing the parts of the brain stem that control breathing and heartbeat. Brain-stem herniation was a known complication of encephalitis. It was rare, and extremely serious; death, or permanent disability, was usually the result.

The man's death, four weeks after the operation that was supposed to have saved his life, provided investigators with an important clue. Encephalitis could be caused by viruses; that would explain why antibiotics, which only affect bacteria, had not reduced the patients' fevers. Only a few families of viruses affect the brain directly. Pathologists at Emory and the CDC examined the man's brain tissue, looking for indications of which virus might be the culprit. Using a special stain, they found antibodies to flaviviruses, a group of viral diseases including yellow fever, dengue, and Japanese encephalitis that are carried by mosquitoes.

Yellow fever had been eliminated in the United States. Dengue was rare outside of Puerto Rico and Texas. But in late summer 2002, there was one mosquito-borne flavivirus that was circulating widely in the southern United States. Doctors for the other three patients checked hurriedly for any confirmatory evidence.

The blood of the heart and liver recipients, and the spinal fluid of the heart recipient and the other kidney-transplant patient, showed antibodies to West Nile virus.

———

West Nile virus was not a new disease organism: It had been discovered in 1937 in Uganda and over sixty years had caused outbreaks in Africa, the Middle East, and Europe. It was mosquito-borne, with a complex life cycle. Certain species of the insects passed the virus to birds; the virus multiplied in the birds' systems and was passed back to other species of mosquitoes when they bit the birds. Those mosquitoes bit humans in turn, passing the disease along to them.

The virus was new to the United States, though. It had made its first appearance in New York City in August 1999. No one knew how it had arrived in the country: in an insect lurking inside an airliner, in the bloodstream of a smuggled exotic bird, or in an unknowingly infected human. Its advent was so unanticipated that the CDC misidentified it at first. They ignored a zoo pathologist's complaints of a widespread die-off of crows and exotic birds, and misdiagnosed cases of illness in humans as St. Louis encephalitis, a related disease. When the bird and human cases were linked and the right pathogen identified, the CDC's scientists were stunned. They had worried for years about mosquito-borne diseases such as malaria infiltrating the country. West Nile virus had not even been on the list of the organisms they feared.

In its first summer in the United States, sixty-two people in greater New York were hospitalized with West Nile. Seven of them died. Experts in arboviral diseases—neurological conditions carried by mosquitoes, ticks, and fleas—expected it to take off with a vengeance the following year when the mosquito season of 2000 arrived. Instead, it simmered. In birds, it spread north as far as the border between New York state and Canada, and south as far as north-central North Carolina. It sickened twenty-one people and killed two. But if the virus was gentle in 2000, it made up for it in 2001. Without warning, it leapfrogged across several states, showed up in July in rural north Florida, and shortly afterward killed an elderly woman who lived near downtown Atlanta. By the end of the year, it had made sixty-six people ill, killing nine of them, and had advanced to the banks of the Mississippi River.

The CDC waited for the summer of 2002 with tense expectation. In three years, the virus had demonstrated both its lethality and its unpredictability. It was expected to make a dash across the country when the mosquito season began in mid-summer.

When the season began, the virus did not just move; it exploded. Over the July 4th holiday, the first case was found on the other side of the Mississippi, in a seventy-eight-year-old man in Louisiana. Within a month, there were seventy-one cases in Louisiana, and five deaths. Within two months, as the transplant-associated cases were unfolding in Atlanta, there were 737 cases in twenty-nine states. Thirty-five of the victims died.

The CDC threw the new EIS officers at the unfolding epidemic. More than forty of them left Atlanta in rapidly dispatched staggered teams. They went to Louisiana, where 205 people had been diagnosed by Labor Day. In the small towns north of Lake Pontchartrain, scientists from the CDC's Colorado arboviral laboratories were struggling to define the true size of the epidemic by searching for patients with unrecognized mild illness. They were sent to Illinois, where the summer's second outbreak took hold in late August; with 165 people sick, many of them senior citizens, the political leadership of Chicago was engaged in fierce discussions over whether to risk the potential environmental damage of mosquito spraying. Two separate groups were sent to Mississippi, where spraying had already started because 104 people fell sick before the end of August. One group walked door-to-door, politely asking residents to donate blood samples that would allow the CDC to estimate an accurate local rate of infection. Another group asked for urine samples, to determine whether residents were being harmed by pesticide spraying.

John Watson, the family practitioner with the shaved head and the Alaska clinic experience, had asked to be assigned to Chicago for his EIS years. He had had barely two weeks to acclimate to the claustrophobic confines of the Cook County Board of Health's strangely shaped building, a windowless torus with pie-shaped offices barely six feet wide, when "a wave broke over the top," he said. Instantly he was plunged into helping his supervisors answer the city council's urgent questions: whether to spray to reduce the mosquito population, even though fresh mosquitoes would hatch in two weeks; or whether to put pesticides down the sewers when there were 3,400 miles of sewers in the city. Every day, the state public health lab called with lists of the patients who had tested positive for West Nile. His task was finding out everything else about the patients—what their symptoms were, who their doctors were, how long they had been hospitalized, and whether they had any risk factors such as age that would put them at extra risk—as a way of defining the outbreak as it developed.

Kirsten Ernst, the nurse who had just completed two master's degrees, was hearing the same plaintive questions in Mississippi. She had been sent out on August 10 as the case counts started to climb. She was in charge of the "red team," the group taking blood samples. (The group collecting urine to check pesticide exposure levels called themselves the "gold team" in response.) As a nurse, she was particularly concerned with the patients' experience. It gave her special insight into the human cost of West Nile.

"Some people had rash and some didn't. Some people had fever, some didn't. It was completely unpredictable," she said. "I had one gentleman who was probably in his late thirties; even three weeks after he got sick, he was so weak that he could barely stand."

Her concern for how victims were feeling became acute when one of her colleagues became her patient. Tracy Creek, a pediatrician from Colorado who wore strings of African beads and dyed her short hair Kool-Aid orange, came out in mid-August in a second wave of EIS officers. They tromped from house to house in Jackson, Mississippi's semitropical heat in one of the wettest summers on record, taking blood samples, administering physicals, and touring property with homeowners to find places where mosquitoes might be breeding. After several weeks, Tracy began to feel ill. She had a fever and a headache. She was tired. Her neck hurt. Abruptly, she could not tolerate light.

Her teammates feared she had contracted West Nile encephalitis, the most serious form of the disease. They talked several times a day to their Atlanta supervisors. They drew her blood and sent it to Colorado, and then helped her on a plane to Atlanta, with a classmate for an escort. By the time she arrived, the first round of tests had come back: negative for West Nile virus infection. At the CDC, her blood was drawn several more times: still negative. She had all the signs and symptoms of West Nile, but no laboratory evidence of infection.

Over several weeks, she recovered. It left her classmates wondering how reliable the tests were, and how much they were placing themselves at risk.

———

The epidemic was moving west, but the nexus of concern stayed focused on Atlanta. All four of the transplant patients had West Nile virus. But where had they gotten it, and when? And why had they become so sick?

Three of the four patients had developed encephalitis. That was against the known odds. Based on the spread of the virus since 1999, the CDC estimated that most people infected with the mosquito-borne organism would never show symptoms. One out of five might have a mild flu-like illness, with fever, achiness, and headache, sometimes accompanied by a rash. One out of 150 would develop the high fever, stiff neck, and sensitivity to light that signaled encephalitis, swelling of the brain, or meningitis, inflammation of the covering of the brain and spinal cord. Of those with serious symptoms, one in ten would be likely to die. Those who died were usually older than sixty-five.

Here though were four patients all seriously ill, one of them dead, and three of them younger than sixty-five. There was a logical explanation for the seriousness of their illness: They were all taking the immune-system-suppressing drugs necessary to keep their bodies from rejecting their transplants. Any infection that took hold in their systems was likely to progress quickly to its most extreme manifestations.

The more difficult question was how they had become infected in the first place. There was no way to tell in the laboratory whether their diseases all came from the same source. Unlike foodborne bacteria, or viruses such as HIV, West Nile does not have divergent strains; all the viral specimens analyzed in U.S. laboratories since 1999 had virtually identical molecular fingerprints. With microbiology unable to help, it was necessary to look epidemiologically for some common factor—and what all four patients had in common was the accident victim from whom their new organs had come. But she had shown no signs of West Nile infection. When her family was consulted about her wish to be an organ donor, they had said that she was well, and none of the tests done before her organs were transplanted had contravened that. Besides, there had never been any evidence that West Nile virus could be passed from person to person, in either the New World or the old. Over four summers, every recorded case in America had been caused by a mosquito bite.

The obvious hypothesis was that the four transplant patients could have been infected naturally. By the beginning of August, West Nile virus infection had been diagnosed in birds, horses, or humans in the Atlanta area and in parts of Florida. The patients could have been exposed before they checked into the hospital; the two kidney recipients, who had both been discharged, might have been bitten once they had gone home.

The math of West Nile virus infection supported the hypothesis. The incubation period of West Nile—the time that elapses between the virus entering the body and the first evidence of symptoms—is three to fourteen days; the four patients had begun to show symptoms from seven to seventeen days after their transplants. The timing matched in a second way as well. It takes at least fourteen days from the time of infection for the markers of the body's immune response—IgM antibodies, those produced when the immune system recognizes that it has never encountered a particular disease organism before—to rise to detectable levels. It was IgM antibodies that the investigators had found in the three surviving patients' blood, in tests that had been done between twenty and twenty-seven days after their operations.

The investigators experienced a brief moment of relief. The dates of operations, symptoms, and tests showed that the four patients could conceivably have been infected by mosquitoes immediately after their transplants. Their infections might turn out to be an exceedingly unlucky coincidence.

Then a piece of information emerged that shattered all their assumptions. Florida's investigators discovered that the heart recipient, a Cuban émigré named Elio Coro, had not checked into the hospital just before his transplant: He had been there for a month already, in the end stages of congestive heart failure.

The lapse of time since he had been outdoors was more than twice the maximum West Nile virus incubation period. The only place he could have acquired the infection was within the walls of Jackson Memorial Hospital, but there was little chance that he had been bitten by a virus-carrying mosquito while confined to a hospital bed and tethered to supplemental oxygen.

The investigators turned back to the organ donor. She was the only remaining link.

Whenever a patient is treated in a hospital, blood samples are taken, primarily to check for blood type in case a transfusion is needed. Leftovers are usually frozen, a just-in-case move that allows doctors to look back and interpret what was going on in a patient's system at the time of hospital admission. ER staff had taken those routine samples from the accident victim when she was brought into the emergency department; more samples had been taken, for reference and record keeping, when she was declared brain-dead and after her organs had been removed for transplant. They were all in Emory's freezers. They were pulled out and double-checked.

The first set of samples, collected on July 30, were clean: No antibody to West Nile virus. The second set, taken July 31, were clean as well. The third set, taken on August 1 as the young woman's organs were harvested, were not.

Like the others, they did not show West Nile virus antibodies; they supplied no evidence that the organ donor was one of the many who are infected with the virus but never exhibit symptoms. What they did show was far more troubling. In her blood, the CDC's lab found nucleic-acid sequences that matched the RNA of West Nile virus. That discovery did not indicate whether the virus was intact and infectious, so a second test was performed. That test, a viral culture, confirmed what investigators had feared: It grew intact West Nile virus from her blood.

The evidence was incontrovertible. The organ donor had had West Nile virus in her system; it had traveled via her blood or organs to the four people who had received them. For the first time on record, West Nile virus had been passed from person to person.

The implications were chilling. On the day of the lab findings, there were more than 850 cases of West Nile virus illness in the country. They represented only the tip of an iceberg, the one-out-of-150 sick enough to seek a doctor's help. If the CDC's estimates of West Nile's prevalence were correct, more than 120,000 Americans might be infected with West Nile and not know it. A certain number of them were likely to give blood.

Blood banks did not possess a test that could identify West Nile virus in donated blood. Until now, there had been no need for one. The procedures the CDC had used to find the virus in the organ donor's blood samples were delicate and expensive and took several days to perform. There was no way they could be used on the millions of units of blood already in the system, or the thousands more that would be donated in West Nile-infested areas before mosquito season ended. The national blood supply was at risk.

The discovery of the virus in the organ donor's blood had an additional troubling implication. West Nile virus multiplies in the body for only a few days after infection; it is at its peak by the time symptoms develop and by the time antibodies rise to measurable levels can no longer be detected. That meant that the young woman had been infected very recently. The question was, how recently? Had she been bitten by a mosquito in the days immediately before her accident, causing an infection that was too new for anyone in her family to have noticed?

The investigators made a final check: They returned to the first and second samples of her blood to look for West Nile virus RNA. If the accident victim had been infected just before she entered the hospital, the nucleic acids would show up in all three sets of blood samples.

They did not. The first set of samples, and the second, contained no West Nile nucleic acids. Only the third set, taken after the massive transfusions that doctors had poured into her, showed the telltale genetic sequence. There was only one possible conclusion. The accident victim had not only passed the virus on to others via her blood or organs; she had received it the same way. One of the units of blood intended to save her life had infected her with West Nile virus immediately before she died.

And some of that blood donation might remain in some blood bank's freezer, ready to infect someone else.

———

In Atlanta, the focus of the investigation shifted. Though Martha had nominally been in charge, many of the tasks so far had been bench work, lab tests coordinated by the CDC and performed by the agency division in Fort Collins that handled insect-borne diseases. The second phase of the investigation, though, was solidly in the realm of epidemiology: tracking down everyone whose blood might have been given to the organ donor, and ascertaining whether they had ever suffered from unrecognized West Nile virus.

It was a mammoth task. The accident victim had received thirty-one units of packed red blood cells, each slightly less than a pint in volume; seventeen units of frozen plasma, the liquid portion of blood; five units of platelets, cells that help the blood to clot; and ten doses of a component that would encourage her blood to clot and slow down bleeding. Some of the transfusions were pooled products, meaning that they included blood components from more than one donor. When the trail was traced back through medical records and blood collection agencies, it revealed the young woman had received blood from sixty-three different donors. The sixty-three donors lived in eight different states. In all eight states, West Nile virus was circulating freely.

And there was more blood to track down. The sixty-three donations had been broken down into 140 blood components: red cells, white cells, platelets, plasma, clotting factors, and antibodies. Almost half of them had gone to the accident victim. It was necessary to find the rest.

The CDC put the word out to the Food and Drug Administration and to blood banks in the South: Every blood component associated with the organ donor must be withdrawn from circulation immediately. For thirty-five of the components, the investigators were too late. They had already been transfused into someone else. That made the next step even more imperative: The investigators would have to figure out which of the sixty-three blood donations had carried the virus.

"By the time we found this out," Martha said, "it was probably two months after most of these people had donated. It made it very complicated."

The investigators decided on a two-pronged approach: They would track down both the blood and the blood donors. Whatever blood they found would be analyzed for the presence of the virus. Whatever donors could be identified—through the blood industry's screen of medical privacy—would be interrogated about their health. Neither effort guaranteed any success. Given the amount of blood that had already been used, the chances of finding enough samples to test were slim. Given the small number of donors, the probability that anyone had been seriously ill was not significant; given the time that had elapsed since their blood was taken, the possibility that they would remember being mildly ill was not great.

But the need to find something was critical. Public and political concern over the state of the blood supply were ratcheting up. On September 5, the CDC announced another West Nile case that might have been caused by a transfusion, one with no connection to the Atlanta accident victim: A twenty-four-year-old Mississippi woman who had a severe postpartum hemorrhage, and got eighteen units of blood, had been hospitalized with meningitis one month later. By

September 20, it had found five more in three more states: one liver transplant, one amputation, one orthopedic surgery, and two chronically ill elderly men who received frequent transfusions. One of the elderly men died.

"The results are not totally conclusive with respect to blood-borne transmission through transfusion," Dr. Jesse Goodman, a deputy director of the FDA, said in a press conference announcing the additional cases. "It is most prudent to assume that blood-borne transmission likely has occurred, at least in some of these instances."

On the day the new cases were announced, there were 1,641 cases of severe West Nile virus illness in thirty-six states and Washington, D.C. Eighty people had died. If blood-borne transmission of West Nile was a reality, the probability that it would happen more frequently was increasing.

———

EIS veterans joked that the acronym really stood for "Everyday I sit." At the Georgia public health unit, Martha was discovering the truth behind the sarcasm.

The division's epidemiology section occupies the fourteenth floor of the state office building, an undistinguished tall monolith in the heart of Atlanta's old downtown. The building, 2 Peachtree Street, looms over an intersection known as Five Points that serves as the city's zero milepost; buildings running north on Peachtree take their street numbers from their distance from the intersection instead of from cross streets. Immediately behind the state building lies the station that serves the crossing of Atlanta's two subway lines. The building is surrounded by fast-food joints, loans-until-payday storefronts, and street vendors hawking goods to commuters. There are usually also a few lost-looking tourists who have not yet realized the city's museums and music venues are more than a mile to the north.

Martha's perch above the cityscape was a soft-walled, dull pink temporary office, part of a cubicle farm that filled the northwest corner of the floor. The cubicle was piled with stacks of paper and notepads and Post-its full of names and phone numbers. The phone, and email, were turning out to be her chief scientific tools. They were how she was tracking down both the donated blood and the blood donors.

Finding the blood turned out to be the less complicated part. Since the early days of the AIDS epidemic twenty years before, when hemophiliacs had unknowingly been given HIV-infected blood, the blood-donation industry had developed elaborate tracking and trace-back systems. Every donation and every product made from it was bar-coded and entered in databases shared by the blood banks and the institutions who bought blood from them. There was an additional check as well. When a pint of whole blood was taken from a donor, the collection agency clamped off a section of the tubing leading from the donor's arm to the bag. When the blood was sent on to be processed, the tubing was supposed to be preserved and frozen. It was called a "retention segment."

Retention segments were not perfect samples for analysis. Despite their name they were not always retained; when they were, they were not necessarily handled perfectly. And they were tiny: They held only 1 cubic centimeter, less than a quarter-teaspoon of blood. After scouring their records, the blood collection agencies in the eight states where the donor blood had been collected were able to find retention segments for only forty-one of the sixty-three donors. The samples were collected and rushed by overnight mail to the Colorado lab. A second pass through the blood banks uncovered the fate of the forty-one blood components that had not yet been transfused into patients. Two had been used up in processing; twelve had been thrown away or broken. Twenty-seven, though, were still intact in hospital and blood-bank freezers. They were yanked from the shelves and sent to Colorado as well.

The second phase of the investigation was more complicated. It involved tracking down the donors—with the blood agencies as intermediaries, because only the agencies had the records that could connect the bar-coded designations on a bag of blood cells with the name and address of the person who had donated them. Because only the collection agencies knew who they were, only the agencies could contact them. Martha, and the CDC investigators, could only specify what they wanted the collection agencies to do.

They decided to check for infection several different ways. The donors would be asked to complete a questionnaire, asking whether they had had West Nile symptoms—fever, headache, sensitivity to light—around the time that they donated blood. Then they would be asked to give a second blood sample. There was no point checking those samples for viral RNA, since any virus would have left the victims' bodies months ago. But the investigators could check for antibodies. A positive antibody test would confirm that, at some point, the donors had been infected with West Nile. It could not reveal when—CDC scientists had found IgM antibodies against West Nile in some victims more than a year after their infection—but it would help rule out those who had never been infected at all.

If the investigation worked as the disease detectives hoped, the tests and questionnaire would work like the lenses of a microscope, clicking one by one into successively sharper focus. First the new blood sample would rule out the donors who had never had West Nile. Then the questionnaire would help identify which of the West Nile victims had been infected recently. Finally, the retention segments would reveal whether any of the donors had given blood during the narrow time period when virus was circulating in their blood.

If all those conditions were met, and if the investigators were lucky, the question of the organ donor's infection with West Nile virus would be resolved.

———

They were lucky.

The collection agencies found every one of the blood donors. Fifty-seven of the sixty-three agreed to complete the questionnaires and to come back to give blood for analysis. One of the fifty-seven samples contained IgM antibodies to West Nile virus. Martha checked the finding against the questionnaire responses; the donor reported having had a fever, headache, rash, and pain in the eyes about two weeks before giving blood. The results were suggestive, but they were not perfect. The antibodies revealed that the donor had had West Nile virus disease, and the report of symptoms confirmed that the infection had happened in the summer of 2002. But if the donor was remembering correctly, the infection must have happened several weeks before the blood donation. By the time the blood was donated, the virus should have disappeared from his system.

Martha turned to the CDC's lab results. All forty-one retention segments and all twenty-seven blood components had been tested three different ways: checked for viral RNA and for IgM antibodies to West Nile virus, and cultured to see whether West Nile virus would grow from them. The retention segments returned only negative results. Among the blood components, there was a single positive. One bag of frozen plasma contained the genetic material of West Nile virus.

Martha compared the two lists of results, from the blood collection agencies and the lab. They matched. The pint of plasma containing West Nile virus had been donated by the man who remembered feeling ill early in the summer—the man whose blood had yielded antibody evidence of a West Nile infection sometime in the past year.

She checked one more list, the numeric identifiers of the units of blood that had been given to the organ donor. The man's code was on the list. It was the last code on the list.

"Blood from this donor," she said, "was the very last blood component the organ donor received."

———

The investigators had drawn clear links between the original blood donor, the accident victim who was given his blood, and the chronically ill patients who received her organs, and the virus along with them. They would never be able to prove with 100 percent certainty that the contaminated blood caused the ultimate infections; there would never be a way to demonstrate that the young woman had not also been bitten by a mosquito immediately before her accident. The proof was strong enough though for the blood industry and the FDA. They began collaborative work on a rapid test for West Nile RNA that would be reliable, inexpensive, and portable enough to be used on blood donations. It was needed. By the end of the mosquito season in mid-autumn of 2002, twenty-three people had been infected with

West Nile through blood transfusions, out of 4,156 cases of the disease that year.

The test was developed over the winter, granted an experimental license by the FDA, and deployed to blood collection agencies in July 2003. By the end of that year, it pulled 1,027 blood donations that were positive for West Nile virus out of the blood supply.

FOUR

Smallpox

1972, Bangladesh

THE BOYS OF BANGLADESH had never seen anyone who looked like Jeffrey P. Koplan. The Massachusetts native was very tall and wiry with the build of a runner. He was pale, with ear-length blond hair and a short, full red beard.

Being white and pale and tall and blond was a recipe for being stared at anywhere in South Asia. Koplan had almost gotten used to that. Sometimes he looked away; sometimes he looked back. Once, feeling the weight of the endless inspection, he had subtly edged closer to a man who was staring at him; the man had backed up, never breaking his gaze, until he stumbled and almost fell backward off the edge of a porch.

The children, though, were not content with staring. Koplan had a bad back, and he was a determined exerciser. Every day, he went running in the sodden tropical heat that hung in the heavy growth along the banks of the Ganges. The children would wait for him. They jumped up and down in excitement as he ran by. "Lal mabood!" they shrieked. "Red monkey, red monkey!"

On good days, they waved at him. On bad days, they threw stones. Koplan kept running. It was important to keep on good terms with the children. They were valuable to the work he was doing. They knew everything that went on in every household in their villages. They especially knew where every case of smallpox was.

————

Jeff Koplan had been an EIS officer for five months when he arrived in Bangladesh. He was twenty-seven years old, from a suburb south of Boston, the son of a lawyer who had opted to work in the family retail business. Koplan had attended a local prep school and then gone on to be an English major and premed at Yale.

His mother was responsible, in part, for his being a doctor. She was diagnosed with cancer when he was in high school and died during his last year of college. His aunt and a cousin had had cancer as well. "There was always illness around, relatives being visited in the hospital, people whispering bad prognoses," he said. "Being a physician had a real positive flavor to it. Maybe I thought in some magical way it would protect me."

Koplan also had a role model: the family's pediatrician, a bristling, intimidating man who wore a tweed jacket, maintained a home laboratory, and could have stepped out of a Norman Rockwell print. He was a Harvard Medical School graduate who had volunteered to be an ambulance driver in France early in World War I. When Koplan went off to medical school at Tufts, on the north side of Boston, the doctor gave him a gift: the monocular brass microscope that he had used at Harvard. Koplan treasured it for years.

Koplan had been drawn to medicine first through history—in his teens, he was fascinated by accounts of early surgical achievements and the discovery of the circulation of the blood—and second by science. In high school, he won a scholarship from the National Science Foundation that put him in a lab for the summer to conduct an experiment. The experiment was to administer different drugs to mice, drop them into a tank of water, and record how well and how fast they swam. It was a goofy-sounding trial—he called himself a "mouse life-guard"—but it taught him how to conduct an experiment and gave him a taste of lab work. He worked in a lab every summer after that, in Boston and once in England, and wrote several papers that were published in medical journals before he graduated from college.

At Tufts, Koplan met his future wife, who was studying pediatrics, and began working with groups that provided health care for the poor. He spent a summer living in Mexico and commuting across the border to a California clinic run by the United Farm Workers. After he had been two years at Tufts, his wife won a slot in a child psychiatry residency in New York City, and he transferred to Mount Sinai School of Medicine in Manhattan. Mount Sinai was the med school for the City University of New York and was known for its programs in community medicine. He found a clinic job in Spanish Harlem.

Koplan started his last year of med school in 1969. It was a year of ferment: of Woodstock, Stonewall, the Manson murders, and the first steps on the moon. It was also the year that the My Lai massacre in Vietnam became public. Opposition to the war had been building steadily—in 1968, a week of antiwar demonstrations shut down Columbia University, a few blocks north of Mount Sinai on the opposite side of Manhattan—but it broke across the country in 1969. In October, there was a nationwide student strike. In November, a half-million people marched on Washington, D.C. Fifty-seven percent of Americans told the Gallup polling organization that U.S. troops should be withdrawn within a year. President Richard Nixon pleaded on TV for the support of "the great silent majority of my fellow Americans."

Koplan had protested the war, but like every other man of his age, he was subject to the draft—unless, as a doctor, he chose some form of national service to compensate. Two of his professors had mentioned the CDC to him. In the spring of 1970, a CDC delegation came to see the Harlem project where he worked. In it was Dr. Phillip Brachman, who had just become chief of the division that housed the Epidemic Intelligence Service. That sealed the deal. Koplan applied to the EIS, was accepted, and agreed to start in 1972, after doing two years of residency.

Landing an EIS assignment was a lot like securing a slot in a medical residency program, a process universally known as "match." New members of the EIS interviewed with CDC divisions and listed their top choices; chiefs of the divisions listed which new officers they desired to hire; the EIS management sorted out discrepancies. Koplan had put the smallpox eradication program as his first choice. He matched.

He wanted the job because it offered the chance to participate in making history. Six years earlier, the World Health Organization and the CDC had dedicated themselves to eradicating smallpox, the most feared infectious disease of all time. And he had been impressed by the people in charge. The head of the CDC smallpox unit was Dr. William H. Foege, who had been an EIS officer in 1962, left to become a medical missionary, and then returned. He was considered a hero by epidemiologists for devising the vaccination strategy that had chased smallpox out of West Africa by 1970.

There had been attempts, over years, to eradicate other diseases, especially yellow fever and malaria, but none had succeeded. The effort to eradicate smallpox, though, was closing in on its goal.

"I knew it was time-limited," Koplan said. "It was a unique opportunity to do something exciting. And I wanted to do overseas work, and there was no question that if you worked on smallpox you would go overseas."

He did not, though, at least not at first. The previous October, the Advisory Committee on Immunization Practices (ACIP), a group of researchers and clinicians that helped the CDC formulate vaccination policy, had recommended that routine vaccination of children against smallpox cease in the United States. The recommendation was based on the recent U.S. history with smallpox: There had not been a case of the disease in the country since 1949. There had been three outbreaks in the 1940s, but all had been sparked by people who were infected before they arrived in the United States. And with smallpox diminishing elsewhere in the world, the odds of new importations seemed low.

Plus, recently published research by two CDC doctors had exposed the risks of routine smallpox vaccination. Responding to reports by pediatricians that children had died after being immunized, John M.

Neff and J. Michael Lane of the CDC's smallpox surveillance unit had found that for every million vaccinations there was at least one death, between fourteen and fifty-two life-threatening reactions such as encephalitis and severe skin disorders, and hundreds of minor reactions as well. Overall, they confirmed, six to eight children were dying each year as a result of their smallpox vaccinations.

The recommendation to stop vaccinating was controversial. One of the importation outbreaks, in 1947, had wreaked havoc in New York City. A man from Maine who was on his way home from a vacation in Mexico had stopped in Manhattan because he felt so ill. He died before doctors recognized what was wrong with him; so did one other New Yorker. Twelve others were infected but survived. When news of the cases broke, more than 6 million New York residents stood in line, sometimes for days, so they could be vaccinated. And there had been more recent outbreaks that pointed up the possibilities of reimportation into the United States. In 1970, a German man who had visited Pakistan unknowingly brought smallpox to his hometown of Meschede; before he died, he infected seventeen other people in the hospital where he was treated. Four died. In early 1972, as U.S. physicians began coming to grips with the ACIP recommendation, an Albanian Moslem who was returning from the hajj pilgrimage to Saudi Arabia created an epidemic that rolled across Yugoslavia: 175 cases and thirty-four deaths.

Koplan's first task, as a budding smallpox epidemiologist, was to explain to confused and angry doctors why stopping vaccination was nevertheless a good idea.

"They had a valid argument," he said. "There was still smallpox in Brazil. It was certainly in India and Pakistan and Bangladesh and Afghanistan and lots of countries in Africa. Importation was a legitimate concern."

The counterarguments were that the risks of importation were low; that if a case came into the country, the risk of spread would be limited by the high number of people vaccinated; and that an unvaccinated person could be protected by being immunized after exposure, if the authorities moved quickly enough. Adding weight on that side of the argument were the serious adverse reactions that Lane and Neff had recorded. The risks of vaccine complications became much harder to justify if the benefit of protection from smallpox became no longer necessary.

For months, Koplan spent most of his time articulating that risk-benefit equation to physicians and medical-school researchers. He answered phone calls. He wrote letters. Frequently, he was sent out from Atlanta to give lectures explaining the decision. When his supervisor, Foege's classmate Dr. Stanley O. Foster, came to him with the possibility of a different assignment—running a controlled clinical trial of a potential smallpox treatment—he jumped at the chance.

In December 1972, he landed in Bangladesh.

———

In all of human history, there had been no other disease like smallpox. It was vicious: It killed at least a third of those infected, and scarred or blinded most of the survivors. It was fast-moving, traveling everywhere that men had gone, carried by armies and traders and missionaries and slaves. It was relentless, roaring up into periodic epidemics, but never fully disappearing in between.

And it had always been there. The written records of its assaults on humanity went back more than three thousand years. Over the centuries, smallpox had devastated cities, changed the course of battles, and stalled the growth of empires. It had shuffled the leadership of dynasties like a pack of playing cards, decimating the royal houses of England, Holland, France, and Austria and killing rulers in India, China, and Japan.

Above all, smallpox was horrible. It puffed the skin out into thousands of pustules that grew and hardened and merged together. The pustules clustered on the face and hands and feet, and pebbled the mouth and throat and rectum. The disease made it impossible to eat or drink or speak, but it left its victims conscious. They were aware of what was happening to them, and of how they would be changed if they survived.

"The smallpox was always present," Thomas Babington Macaulay wrote in his mid-nineteenth-century *History of England,* "filling the churchyard with corpses, tormenting with constant fear all whom it had not yet stricken, leaving on those whose lives it spared the hideous traces of its power." He called it "the most terrible of all the ministers of death."

Centuries of experience had taught people what to expect from smallpox. High fever was the first sign, along with a splitting headache and vivid dreams. At that point, though victims did not know it, they had already been infected for at least ten days. After three more days, the fever subsided, leaving victims feeling deceptively well but with a characteristic involuntary look of anxiety. Then a faint rash would appear: inside the mouth first, then on the face and limbs, and then on the trunk. Within twenty-four hours, it covered the body. Then it began to change: The flat red spots pushed above the skin and filled with fluid that shimmered faintly and then took on the dull yellow opacity of pus. The pustules grew and stretched, ripping the epidermis away from the underlying structure of the skin; when they were touched, they felt hard under pressure and could be rolled under the skin like a piece of metal shot. At their worst, ten days after the rash appeared, they developed a faint dimpling at the apex; then they subsided slowly as the body reabsorbed their contents. At two weeks, the sores began to scab over; at three weeks, the scabs fell off, leaving a pale, shallow scar. Victims were infectious from before the rash appeared until the scabs fell off, and the scabs by themselves could transmit the disease once they separated from the body.

That was the classic form of smallpox, caused by a virus named *Variola major*. There was a lesser form, *Variola minor,* with a milder rash and a lower death rate. And there were more frightening forms, also caused by variola major but occurring infrequently: flat smallpox, which almost always occurred in children, in which the fever never abated and the lesions sank into the skin and became bloody; and hemorrhagic pox, which struck only adults, caused bleeding and bruising so severe that skin came to resemble purple suede, and killed its victims within six days.

Reliable protection against smallpox was sought for centuries. The most successful attempt was a practice called variolation, which introduced pus from smallpox sores into small cuts in the skin. If it worked, variolation protected against the disease, but it carried a high risk of causing full-blown smallpox that could be passed to others. Edward Jenner, an English country doctor, made the practice safe in 1796. Taking note of a longtime folk belief that milkmaids who got cowpox, a mild pustular disease of cattle, never contracted smallpox, he cut the arm of an eight-year-old boy named James Phipps and inserted some pus taken from a milkmaid's hand. Two weeks later, he repeated the procedure, using smallpox pus to guarantee that the boy would be infected. Phipps never developed the disease.

Jenner called his variant technique of using a mild disease to protect against a deadly one "vaccination," from the Latin word for cow. It was resisted at first, and then spread rapidly through Europe and the Americas. Over 100 years, it began to force smallpox out of the human population. By 1895, there was no smallpox in Sweden; the disease vanished from Austria by 1920 and from Russia sometime in the 1930s. By the 1960s, health authorities began to hope that a wish expressed by Jenner in 1801 could be achieved, that "this practice would wipe out this scourge from the face of the earth."

Unique circumstances made that possible. Smallpox, it turned out, infected only humans. Though there were many related diseases that affected animals, there was no animal reservoir where smallpox itself could hide. Smallpox infection also gave a survivor lifelong immunity against contracting smallpox again, which meant that a vaccination campaign would have to reach not the entire human population—an impossible task—but only those still vulnerable. Vaccination against smallpox had been proved over 170 years to reliably break the person-to-person chain of smallpox transmission. And because smallpox was so loathesomely distinctive, its remaining reservoirs were not hard to find.

There were many. In 1966, when the World Health Organization (WHO) made smallpox eradication an international priority, the disease was circulating freely in thirty-three countries and intermittently in eleven more. The previous year, 131,000 cases had been recorded, but health authorities suspected there were 100 times that many.

By late 1972, most smallpox cases were in six countries: Botswana, Ethiopia, Nepal, Pakistan, India, and Bangladesh. The situation in

Bangladesh was dire. In December 1971, the country had finally achieved independence, shedding its former label of East Pakistan after a brutal civil war. Between August 1970 and the proclamation of nationhood, it had not had a single smallpox case. Once independence was declared, though, more than 10 million refugees who had fled from the fighting into India streamed back across the borders.

They brought smallpox with them. In Atlanta, a CDC staff member saw a TV newscast of the huge migration, and spotted the unmistakable pustules of smallpox on members of the crowd. In mid-1972, the CDC sent Foster to Dhaka to try to reestablish control of the situation. By the end of the year, he estimated there were 70,000 cases of smallpox in Bangladesh.

———

There had never been a successful treatment for smallpox. Over the centuries, many had been tried. All the methods were based on the notion that illness signaled an imbalance in the body, and all of them failed.

Smallpox patients were purged, with laxatives and emetics. They were bled, using leeches that attached to the skin or small blades to cut slits into veins. They were made to sweat, wrapped in thick blankets and parked in front of roaring fires; or "cupped" with glass vessels that were heated before being placed on the skin, so that they would form a vacuum as they cooled and suck the flesh under them up into welts; or blistered with chemicals and hot metals. Some doctors tried to banish the disease by cooling its intense fever. They made victims sleep without blankets under open windows, or wrapped them in bandages drenched in cold water, or allowed them to eat only "cooling" foods such as oatmeal and fruit. Some administered botanical concoctions such as cinchona bark, the source of quinine, because it was known to reduce the fever of malaria. In Europe, royal patients were wrapped in red cloth and kept in rooms with red hangings, on the theory that the color would warm the body and encourage blood to rush to the skin.

Where treatments failed, divine intercession was sought. In Europe, the image of Saint Nicaise, a fifth-century bishop of Rheims who survived an attack of smallpox only to be beheaded by the Huns a year later, was worn on protective amulets. The Chinese had a smallpox goddess who was believed to send the disease in order to mar the appearance of attractive children. When a child came down with the pox, family members would make daily offerings in the goddess's temples, hoping to persuade her to keep the attack mild so the child would not be disfigured. In West Africa, there was a smallpox god, whose priests collected smallpox victims' scabs to use for inoculations.

The most influential deity, the one whose worship stretched the farthest and lasted the longest, was Shitala Mata, the Hindu goddess of smallpox. She was venerated throughout southeast Asia in a cult that began before the common era and persisted through the smallpox eradication campaign. Her name meant "the cooling one." People prayed to her to keep smallpox from their families, or to make an attack a mild one. When smallpox came anyway, it was believed to be sent by the goddess. The vaccination campaign ran into great difficulty in areas where worship of Shitala was strong, particularly in the very poor Indian states on the border of Bangladesh. To accept vaccination, worshipers felt, was to defy Shitala's will.

The late nineteenth-century discoveries of the germ theory and of the existence of bacteria and viruses did nothing to dislodge belief in smallpox deities, but they did destroy trust in dietary and humoral treatments for smallpox. They also failed to substitute any useful solutions. As antibiotics were developed, starting with penicillin in 1940, they were tried against smallpox without success; they could protect against secondary bacterial infections that might follow the pustules, but could do nothing to affect the virus. The emergence of antiviral drugs in the 1970s, as the eradication campaign was proceeding, offered some hope of forestalling the disease—if they could be proven to work, produced in a volume to make them profitable, and delivered to the Third World, where most of the remaining cases of smallpox were clustered, all possibilities that seemed dubious. The smallpox eradicators were both intrigued by the possibility of anti-smallpox drugs—smallpox remained an incurable disease with a 20 to 40 percent mortality rate—and also worried about them. If nations acquired a drug that could cure smallpox, the international effort to eradicate the disease would lose most of its reason for existing just as it was nearing its goal.

The drug that the CDC wanted Koplan to test was a new antiviral called adenine arabinoside, Ara-A for short. In animal and human trials, it had shown some effect on herpes and cytomegalovirus infections. It also had worked against vaccinia, the virus used in the smallpox vaccine. Since the two viruses were so similar, investigators hoped Ara-A would work against smallpox as well. Ara-A was a reformulation of a similar compound, cytosine arabinoside or Ara-C, that a Bangladeshi doctor living in Canada named M. S. Hossain had reported using on smallpox victims. Eight of his nine patients had recovered, but it was not known whether the drug had helped; the group was too small to draw any conclusions from.

Foster proposed that Koplan conduct a full scientific trial—randomized, controlled, and blinded—of the new compound, Ara-A. The experiment needed to be conducted where smallpox was naturally occurring. Bangladesh had volunteered an empty ward in its infectious diseases hospital in the capital, Dhaka, and Parke-Davis had agreed to supply the drug. All that was needed was everything else: IVs, syringes, bags of fluid, lab equipment, tubes and slides, microscopes and technicians. Running a clinical trial was more complicated than merely giving the drug to patients and watching whether they survived or died. It required taking vital signs, drawing and analyzing blood, recording EKGs, and running viral cultures, for every patient, several times a day.

Koplan began gathering the equipment, begging donations from major manufacturers. Over three months, he accumulated almost two tons' worth in an Atlanta warehouse. Then there was the problem of lab staff. He was going to an unfamiliar hospital, with no time to evaluate the abilities of anyone who might be working there. Instead, he decided to do the work himself. He began spending a few hours a day in the CDC's hematology lab, practicing analysis of blood chemistries and refreshing skills he had not used since medical school.

The way to administer Ara-A was in an intravenous solution, 20 milligrams of the drug for every kilogram of body weight. The manufacturer sealed the drug and the placebo in coded vials. They gave the code to Koplan in a sealed envelope.

Foster had already moved to Bangladesh, to supervise the eradication program there. Koplan handed over the envelope when he arrived.

———

In medieval Europe, the buildings where the victims of plague and smallpox were taken, ostensibly for treatment but usually merely to die, were called pest houses. The Dhaka Infectious Disease Hospital was a pest house. It was a dank, stained concrete shell in an empty field. Cows grazed around it. Birds landed on the sills of the unglazed windows. Smallpox victims were brought there, and they died.

The ward the authorities had offered was an unused floor of the hospital. Koplan hired cleaners to scrub it and move in the beds and the lab equipment. He found a former sergeant-major from the Pakistani army to handle logistics, some local physicians to evaluate the patients day to day, and a man he met in the market whose job was to make sure the patients were fed. Family members were supposed to take care of hospital patients, but few family members cared to come to the smallpox hospital. Once patients vanished through the doors, they were at risk of starving in their beds. The aide's job was not just buying food for the study subjects; it was cooking it for them and sitting by their beds to spoon-feed them if they were too weak to lift a bowl themselves. Most of them were.

Koplan also found an unanticipated collaborator. Hossain, the Bangladeshi investigator who had conducted the Ara-C study, had returned to the country. Hospital authorities announced to Koplan that they were adding Hossain to the CDC study. He would conduct an Ara-C evaluation, using the same control patients Koplan had enrolled as a gauge for the validity of his study. Their results would be published together.

Koplan was furious, and powerless. The study went ahead.

He evolved a routine: Up at 6:00 a.m. to the local cholera hospital to borrow an EKG machine because the infectious hospital did not own one. Over to the smallpox hospital to take EKGs on every study subject. Back to the cholera hospital with the EKG, carefully cleaned with alcohol so it would not transmit smallpox, and then back to the pest house again to do rounds with the clinical team. Each morning, every patient was checked and photographed to document the progression of the disease. Blood was drawn, vitals were taken, and a new set of IVs were made up and plugged in. The medications and the placebo solution looked different once they were mixed and hung over the beds in the old, thick-walled glass IV bottles, so the clinical team took care of the mixing, and pulled a brown paper bag over the bottle before Koplan came near. Administering the drugs, or the placebo masquerading as one, took eight hours. Late mornings were for doing the blood chemistries. Lunch, when Dhaka shut down, was for exercise. Afternoons and evenings were devoted to examining new patients and admitting them to the study. There were Bengali lessons for two hours every night.

The study took anyone younger than sixty and older than six months, but it excluded women of child-bearing age (because Ara-A might cause birth defects), anyone with an additional illness, and anyone with the most serious form of smallpox, the swift-moving and almost universally deadly hemorrhagic pox. The days leaked into each other, a steady progression of new patients with fever and anxious faces and the inescapable rash that grew until it covered their bodies.

"It was horrible," Koplan said. "You would see someone who had just a light rash, and it would progress and progress until it covered them. And then they died. There are very few things you do in medicine where 25 percent of your patients die, except care of the elderly, and virtually all of our patients were young."

The investigators had enrolled thirty-one patients who met the criteria: eleven controls who received the placebo, and twenty receiving either Ara-A or Ara-C. There were nine young children, a baby, two girls on the verge of menarche; one man in his fifties, and the rest young men. One man killed himself the day after he was brought to the hospital. Of the rest, half developed confluent smallpox: The maturing pustules merged together, tearing the skin away from its underlying layers until it formed a hard, pebbled sheet stretched over a layer of pus. Five developed flat pox: The lesions never formed pustules, but sank into the skin, making dark purple patches with a velvety feeling to them. The patches had a red ring around them; when they were touched, the skin peeled away, leaving weeping raw flesh that resembled a severe burn.

The flat-pox patients died three to five days after they were brought to the hospital. That was expected. But as the study went on, Koplan realized that other patients were dying also, even ones with milder smallpox who should have survived—scarred or blinded, perhaps, but alive. Several patients died when they seemed to be past the danger point, when their lesions were drying up and their temperatures dipping toward normal. Something was wrong.

They were three months into the study. It was early to stop, given the investment they had made, but the death rate made Koplan worried. He persuaded Foster to open the envelope, and break the code.

"When we analyzed the results, we found that there was no difference between the drug I was testing and the placebo," he said. "And the other drug, the cytosine arabinoside, was killing the patients."

By the time they stopped, four of the eleven placebo patients had died, five of the nine Ara-A patients, and nine of the ten receiving Ara-C. The drugs had made no difference. There was still no successful treatment for the most terrible of all the ministers of death.

———

The study was closed down. Koplan returned to Atlanta, to the desk job he had had in the smallpox eradication unit, explaining the decision to end domestic vaccination. He spent a month at Los Angeles County Hospital, assisting in a study of the biology of smallpox vaccine. He also picked up an additional task, fielding calls from doctors near major ports and airports—Chicago, Miami, New York—who had found a case of rash and fever in someone trying to enter the country. Several times a week, usually during dinner, a quarantine officer would call with a case description and a request to send specimens for analysis by CDC's smallpox lab. Koplan became the middleman, discussing the case with the local doctor, and relaying back lab results from the CDC.

The cases were never smallpox. The nooses cast around the disease by the eradication program had tightened and held. The Bangladesh project, though, proved unexpectedly useful in proving that importation had ceased. Out in the field, Koplan's EIS colleagues were organizing vaccine campaigns and tracking down remaining cases; they could recognize smallpox on sight, but they seldom spent much time with a victim. Koplan, by contrast, had seen a ward full of patients through to death or recovery. It made him one of the few Western doctors of his generation who had taken care of the full clinical spectrum of smallpox, a voice of experience that could be usefully soothing to the uneasy doctors on the other end of the phone.

In 1973, Koplan went back to Bangladesh for three months to do the case-finding side of smallpox work. It reunited him with Stan Foster, who had remained in the country, determined to see the disease through its endgame.

Foster almost did not have the chance. By October 1974, smallpox was confined to only two areas of Bangladesh. But fall was monsoon season: The country was struck with the worst floods in fifty years. Hundreds of thousands of people fled the low-lying areas near the coast and riverbanks, heading for the cities. Three months later, the government destroyed the slums the refugees had created, forcing them to return to their villages with bulldozers at their backs.

Smallpox traveled with them. The disease exploded across the country, unerringly finding the percentage of the population who remained susceptible. The president declared a national emergency. WHO poured staff into the crisis. By November 1975, Foster and his eradicators had not seen a case of smallpox for two months. On November 14, they declared victory over smallpox in Bangladesh.

The next morning, Foster got three telegrams. "One was from the WHO; it said, 'Congratulations,'" he said. "One was from the CDC; it said, 'Great job.' And one was from an eradicator on Bhola Island in the Bay of Bengal. It said, 'We have a case of smallpox.'"

Foster left immediately, catching a ride on an aging paddlewheel steamer, unironically called *The Rocket,* that had been beating the same route up and down the Ganges for more than fifty years. It took eight hours to go the one hundred miles to Bhola, in the Ganges Delta.

When he arrived, the local eradicators walked him to a house well inland, where he found a three-year-old girl named Rahima Banu. She was already recovering; the pustules had dried up and crusted over. They scoured the island, but found no other cases. Rahima was the last naturally occurring case of variola major left in the world.

Before they left the island, Foster took some of the scabs from the girl's sores, and kept them. He sent them on to the CDC before leaving for his next assignment in smallpox's remaining hot spot, Somalia. The last occurrence of variola minor was found in a Somali named Ali Maow Maalin in October 1977.

Foster met Rahima Banu again in Bangladesh in 2000; she had married and had three children. Her virus lives on as well. Poxvirus scientists at the CDC cultured it from her scabs, and kept it. It exists, along with several hundred others, in a freezer in a protected, undisclosed location at the CDC in Atlanta. After the WHO declared in 1980 that smallpox had been eradicated worldwide, it began consolidating every existing sample of virus into two repositories, at the CDC and in Russia. They remain the only known, legal stocks of smallpox virus in the world.

Whether other stockpiles exist, in the hands of terrorists or the labs of rogue nations, is still unknown.

FIVE

Listeriosis

August–November 2002,
Philadelphia

IT BEGAN WITH THREE BABIES.

It was the middle of August. The babies, who were not related, had been born in the previous two weeks in towns in the western part of Pennsylvania. They were not well. Their doctors had run tests and ordered cultures. Independently, each had made the same discovery: The babies had an illness called listeriosis.

Listeriosis is a foodborne disease, caused by a bacterium called *Listeria monocytogenes*. It is rare, and difficult to track because weeks can elapse between infection and the start of symptoms. But it is also a dangerous disease, particularly to the elderly and ill, and to women who are pregnant.

Listeria was so troublesome that Pennsylvania had recently imposed a new rule: All cases of listeriosis must be reported to the state health department. The report of the three babies' cases came in to the state department, and then, because it was August and people were on vacation, was handed to the Philadelphia Department of Public Health, where EIS officer Claire Newbern had just settled in to her new job.

Claire was a Ph.D. epidemiologist whose specialty was the ways that race, class, and income affect health. She had done her dissertation on how family structure and education affected the prevalence of sexually transmitted diseases among teenagers, and had asked to work in Philadelphia because a city was a perfect laboratory for studying what she was interested in.

The listeriosis outbreak looked small to begin with, and then it did not. On August 21, the Pennsylvania Department of Health sent an email to all the counties in the state, asking their health departments to check for other cases of listeria. By August 23, Claire had ten additional cases. By August 30, she had a total of twenty-two, and two people had died. Because listeriosis had only just become a reportable disease, the records for past years were incomplete—but they seemed to indicate that, in most years, Pennsylvania saw eight to ten cases of listeria. Claire had more than twice that many, with four months of the year to go.

"It was building and building, and we realized we needed help," she said. "We agreed we needed to call the CDC."

The agreement between the CDC and state health departments regarding where EIS members are going and what they are supposed to investigate is set out in a document called an Epi-Aid Memorandum. Over the years, the deployments had taken on the name of the document. The investigation of listeria cases in Pennsylvania was the 2002 fiscal year's Epi-Aid 73.

The day after Pennsylvania formally asked for help, a CDC team arrived in Philadelphia: Claire's classmate Sami Gottlieb, a master's-degree epidemiologist named Nicole Baker, and a veterinary medical student named Michelle Jefferson who was spending an elective semester at the CDC. Because it was so soon after EIS training, a second-year officer came with them: Andi Shane, a physician. It was expected that Shane would stay a few days, to get them started. After that, Sami Gottlieb would be in charge.

Sami was thirty-six, an internal medicine physician who had already taught medical students and done public health research before she came to the EIS. She was from Prairie Village, Kansas, a town of 22,000 people that was a suburb of Kansas City. She was the oldest; she had a brother and sister who were twins. Despite the bucolic surroundings, their growing-up had been hard. Their parents divorced when Sami was ten, and three years later their mother was diagnosed with advanced breast cancer. She was thirty-seven. She survived, though she was sick and taking chemotherapy for much of the time Sami was in high school.

Sami left Kansas for college at Stanford University, where she took a seminar with Carl Djerassi, the developer of the birth control pill. Research for the course took her into local high schools where two out of five girls were pregnant or had children. She was already focused on becoming a doctor, but the experience started her thinking about the social and political aspects of health. AIDS had been identified only five years before; Djerassi's students banded together to campaign for condom dispensers in Stanford's dormitories. The effort was controversial, though ultimately successful. "It made such obvious sense," Sami said. "But we received such resistance."

In medical school at University of California-San Francisco, she studied how the homeless used local emergency rooms for health care. In the school's primary care/internal medicine residency, she witnessed the struggle for common ground between academic medicine and managed care.

"Every rotation I did in medical school I thought was interesting: 'Oh, I want to be a hematologist,' 'No, I want to be an obstetrician,'" she said. "But I kept being interested in the bigger picture."

She had heard about the EIS from a friend at UCSF and planned to apply for the summer of 1995, when she finished residency. She had downloaded the application and finished the essay, months early. And then she met Scott Filler. They had seen each other a few times at the gym, and chatted; their first long conversation came in the spring of '95. Shortly afterward, they started going out. He was far behind her in school—finishing his first year, while she was ending her training—but Sami had heard him say he worked in the business world before reorienting toward medicine. She thought they were the same age. He was actually three and a half years younger. He had fudged the history and added a few years to be sure she would go out with him.

Their backgrounds were strikingly different—Scott was a native Californian, easygoing where she fretted over small details—but they were both athletic, committed to medicine, and passionate about travel. To wait out Scott's schooling, Sami traveled for seven months, studying Spanish in South America and then backpacking in Thailand, Nepal, and Vietnam. Then she came back to San Francisco and became an assistant clinical professor at UCSF, seeing patients at a clinic at the San Francisco Veterans' Administration Hospital and supervising medical residents and students.

"After residency, you know a lot of medicine, but you haven't had time to really learn from experience," she said. "So I was glad I did it. But I realized it didn't suit my personality much. I thought about my patients all the time, and worried about them, and called them at home. I was exhausted every night, and feeling like I was looking only at little problems when I wanted to move on to big, complex puzzles."

Within a year, Scott finished school and matched to a residency program in Denver. Sami, who loved San Francisco but wanted to stay with Scott, was unsure whether to go as well. A friend from her residency program mentioned a fellowship that would let her get a public health degree at University of Colorado while working for the Denver Public Health Department. She applied, got in, and spent three years studying sexually transmitted diseases.

"I found out I was a nerd," she said. "I really liked sitting in front of a computer and doing data analysis and applying statistics. I was still able to see patients, but I could see how my research fit into the larger picture, and what policy implications it had."

When Scott finished, it was Sami's turn to choose where they went next. She had never forgotten about the EIS, and the persistence of her interest piqued Scott's curiosity as well. Throughout their training, they had promised each other that they would travel together once they were both done. When the summer of 2001 came, they both mailed in applications, and then left the country. They were in an internet café in Ecuador when they heard they had both been accepted to the class of 2002.

They came back to interview for jobs in April 2002 at the annual EIS conference. They created a small stir: They were the only married couple in the class, they were striking together—Sami with waist-length blond hair, wide blue eyes, and sharp cheekbones, Scott several inches taller, hazel-eyed, and dark—and they were six hours late. They had flown directly from Asia, and their flight had been delayed.

The EIS conference was always in Atlanta, always in the spring, and always busy, because it served several purposes at once. It was a scientific meeting for current corps members who wanted to present accounts of their investigations; it was a reunion opportunity for the tightly knit alumni; and it was a hiring fair. Supervisors looking for new EIS officers wore orange dots or yellow stars on their conference badges—orange for Atlanta postings, yellow for state departments. They trolled the hotel hallways, readying their pitches whenever they spotted the red badges that new recruits were required to wear. By the end of the week, the offices doing the hiring and the new recruits looking for jobs were expected to tell the EIS organizers what their preferences were. It took one more weekend for the match to be worked out. The Monday after the conference, the new class members learned which jobs they would report to in July.

Scott knew what he wanted—his main interest was malaria—but after three years working on STDs, Sami was ready to consider other options. She was aggressively recruited by the Foodborne and Diarrheal Diseases Branch, and she matched.

———

Foodborne, as it is called in CDC shorthand, is one of the largest employers of EIS members: It takes five of every class, so there are ten corps members—five first-years and five second-years—in the branch all the time. It is one of the least specialized postings, since foodborne diseases can be caused by so many different organisms. And it is one of the busiest: There are 76 million cases of foodborne illness in the United States every year.

"It's sort of a liberal arts education in public health, coming to work for us," said Robert Tauxe, the branch chief.

Tauxe was an internist approaching fifty whose thick hair had gone prematurely silver; he sported a formidable mustache and almost always wore a bow tie. He was married to an architect, spoke four modern languages besides English, and labeled his archive of notebooks in Latin. Above the notebooks in his windowless basement office was a shelf of toys and trophies representing the culprits in foodborne outbreak investigations he had supervised: fruit, cheese, sprouts, a chicken, and a small hamburger for a 1993 epidemic that sickened 750 people in Washington, Idaho, California, and Nevada, killed four children, and exposed the dangers of the bacterium E. coli O157.

Tauxe had been an EIS officer in 1983, in the branch that he now headed. Paul Blake, his mentor, had sent him to Mali to work on a stubborn outbreak of cholera. Cholera was usually caused by contaminated water, but water could not be blamed this time as Mali was suffering through a three-year drought. The country was drying out; the Sahara was advancing, covering fields and turning villagers into refugees. The one remaining food was millet, for those who could afford it. Those who could not were eating field grass and weeds. In a twist on the usual expectation that disease falls hardest on the poorest, the cholera victims were the ones who ate the millet, not the ones who had no food at all.

The millet was cooked and shared in big communal vessels; up to twenty people ate with their hands out of a single bowl. Anything left over was put away for the next day. The grain was starchy, moist from cooking, and always warm because the climate was so hot—a perfect growth medium for *Vibrio cholerae,* the bacterial cause of cholera. It was an obvious conclusion; too obvious, Tauxe soon realized, because the refugees had always eaten their millet in this manner, and yet they had only recently been hit by the disease.

He bought some millet to bring back to Atlanta to test. He asked the refugees how to cook it, to be sure he was reproducing their recipe correctly. They thought it charming that a rich American would want to eat their subsistence food, and they explained the preparation carefully. They added, regretfully, that they could not show him the exact right way.

"They said, 'If our goats had enough to eat and drink, they would be making milk, and we would make yogurt from the milk and put it on the millet,' " Tauxe said. "So I brought a sack of millet back, and I searched around Atlanta until I found a herd of Nubian goats, because that was the type of goat in Mali. We made yogurt from the milk. We cooked the millet. We added yogurt to some of the millet, and then we inoculated the millet with yogurt and the millet without it with vibrio. But yogurt is really acidic, and vibrio hates acid. So when we made the millet the traditional way, the cholera just would not grow."

––––––

Listeria, the culprit in the Pennsylvania outbreak, was a newcomer to the group of organisms the foodborne group dealt with. It had been known for decades to be a cause of human illness, but researchers had only recognized in 1981 that it traveled by means of food. Listeriosis is a rare disease: There are only about 2,500 cases a year in the United States, compared to 2.4 million cases of campylobacter and 1.4 million cases of salmonella. It has an incubation period that can stretch from several days to more than a month, making an outbreak much harder to research than staphylococcal food poisoning, which strikes within hours. And listeria has a quirk that is unique among the foodborne bugs: It grows very well in the cold.

"We find it in the intestines of animals, but that's not its real home," Tauxe said. "It's really adapted to places that are way below the body temperature of an animal—moist, dark, cold places, rotting vegetation, damp slimy corners. The advent of refrigeration controlled a lot of other bacteria, but it opened up a little niche for listeria."

It is hard to know how many Americans are exposed to listeria each year, because the bacteria does not cause disease in healthy people. In immunocompromised adults and the elderly, it causes fever, diarrhea, septicemia, and meningitis. It strikes pregnant women with double force, giving them a mild illness but then causing miscarriage or stillbirth. Its viciousness among those groups is the chief reason why the

CDC cares about such a rare disease: Listeria kills one out of every five people who develop serious illness, compared to one in 120 for salmonella or E. coli and one in 1,000 for campylobacter.

Because listeria is so rare, researching it is a particular challenge: There are many sporadic cases, and in most years only a few clusters that can easily be identified as related illnesses. To work through the challenge, the CDC had begun applying molecular biology to the disease. The effort had proved so successful that the laboratory results had begun driving the epidemiology. It was a reversal of the usual pattern in which foodborne investigators found all the cases first, and then brought bacterial isolates from them to the lab for confirmation. With listeria, the lab uncovered the outbreaks, and then told the epidemiologists where to find them.

It worked like this. In 1995, the CDC established a network called PulseNet that linked its foodborne diseases lab with state public health laboratories. The "pulse" in PulseNet stands for pulsed-field gel electrophoresis, or PFGE for short. PFGE is a lab technique that allows precise molecular fingerprinting of bacteria. Operators snip bacterial DNA into pieces using enzymes that are tailored to recognize a particular sequence of nucleic acids. The fragments that result are spread on a gel medium; when electrical currents are run through the medium, the fragments separate and can be compared easily. When fragments from different cases match, that is proof the cases were caused by the same strain of bacteria and belong to the same outbreak.

PFGE is an exacting technique, easily subject to errors; to participate in the network, state laboratories first had to prove they could repeatedly perform the test to CDC standards. Once they qualified, they agreed to do regular fingerprinting for their areas for all cases of illness caused by four organisms: salmonella, shigella, E. coli O157, and listeria. Every PFGE pattern was emailed to an archive at the CDC; together, they made a continually growing database of the major foodborne bugs circulating in the United States.

The database was a crucial tool in characterizing foodborne outbreaks because the distribution of food, and the epidemiology of foodborne disease, had undergone radical change. Before about 1950, a

U.S. foodborne outbreak was likely to be small, localized, and con-fined to people who had something in common—patrons of a restaurant, for instance, or guests at a wedding. By the 1970s, food production had become industrialized. Farms expanded to take in thousands of animals, making it easy for pathogens to circulate among them. Animals from hundreds of farms were trucked to the same slaughterhouses, further increasing the chances that disease organisms could spread. Then meat from the slaughterhouses was sold to conglomerates that were corporate owners for a dozen different supermarket companies operating in different states. Cereal, fruit, and vegetable growers followed the same pattern of concentrated production and widened distribution. The distance between producer and seller, which had protected the consumer against the spread of foodborne disease, collapsed—and grew even more irrelevant after the 1993 signing of the North American Free Trade Agreement, which increasingly brought fruits and vegetables cultivated in other countries into the United States.

Once food distribution changed so markedly, foodborne disease patterns shifted also. In late 1996, epidemiologists in Seattle noticed a small uptick in cases of E. coli O157; in the end, the outbreak took in seventy people, one of whom died, in four states and British Columbia. They had all drunk apple juice made by a single producer from apples processed in one orchard on a single day. Two years later, an outbreak of salmonella sickened 409 people in twenty-three states; it was traced to a single type of toasted-oat cereal manufactured at a plant in Minnesota.

Both times, the far-flung cases of illness were determined to be outbreaks by the molecular fingerprints of the pathogens recovered from the patients: The PFGE patterns were identical even though the patients were separated by hundreds of miles. The technique also linked eighty listeria cases, scattered among twenty-two states, in 1998. That outbreak was first noticed among four people—three adult men and a baby—in Tennessee. PFGE results led investigators to related cases in Ohio, New York, Connecticut, and then Michigan. The outbreak was eventually traced to a hot-dog production line at a Michigan meat processing plant.

Pennsylvania was a newcomer to PulseNet and had not yet tackled listeria. In the last few days of August, Claire collected all of the patients' bacterial isolates and had them FedExed to the CDC. Lewis Graves, the foodborne lab's PFGE specialist, worked over the Labor Day weekend to set up the test. On Monday, he gave a set of gels to Susan Hunter, a senior PulseNet scientist. She spotted a match: Seven of the cases shared an identical DNA fingerprint, a rare one. One day later, there were two more matches: The state labs in New York and Maryland had each found two patients whose PFGE patterns were indistinguishable from the Pennsylvania cases. Wherever the listeria had come from, it was spreading.

———

The goal of a foodborne outbreak investigation is simple: Find the food that is transmitting the disease organism, and take it out of circulation so the disease cannot continue to spread. Simple is not the same as easy. In past outbreaks, listeria had proved it could travel in many foods, including shrimp, soft cheeses, undercooked chicken, hot dogs, raw milk, deli cold cuts, and pate. Before they could figure out which specific item had given the patients listeria, the investigators would have to narrow their inquiry to one type of food.

The CDC called this phase of an investigation "hypothesis generation." Translated from epi-speak, that meant throwing as wide a net as necessary, without making assumptions or prejudging, so that the investigation could be focused in the right direction. The disease detectives needed to move quickly because listeria's long incubation period had stacked the odds against them. Every day that passed reduced the likelihood that those who were infected could accurately remember what they had eaten weeks before. And the outbreak was expanding. The day after they arrived in Philadelphia, it claimed its first death in the city, an elderly man.

Claire and Sami set off to talk to the patients whom the foodborne lab identified as sharing the same PFGE pattern. It was important to confine the questioning to them, since sharing the same bacterial strain made it likely they had been infected in the same manner. To include a patient with a different strain of listeria—about half the patients examined in Pennsylvania so far—risked introducing a confounder, an element that would drag the investigation off-track. Over three days, they trekked across Philadelphia and central Pennsylvania, meeting nine patients including a young male schoolteacher in the suburbs, a Latino grandfather, an elderly couple, and a ninety-eight-year-old retired physician.

They had so little in common, Sami thought. And yet, somewhere in their lives, there had to be something that was the same.

Some of the bacterial isolates collected by the state health department had been held for several weeks before being tested. By the time Claire and Sami met the patients, their initial symptoms were a month in the past. Given listeria's long incubation period, that meant they could have eaten the food that infected them more than two months earlier.

"We did anything we could to help them remember," Sami said. "We had them get calendars, credit card receipts, their checkbooks. We asked them about different events—weddings, Little League games. We walked them through whatever they would eat on a usual day. And then we went through their refrigerators."

The patients were not always willing to help, at first. There was one woman whom the two were eager to talk to. She had been seven months pregnant when she developed listeriosis. It barely made her ill, but it sent her into premature labor, and her son was born at thirty weeks, significantly underdeveloped and very sick. When Claire and Sami found her, he was still hospitalized. They drove up to her apartment in one of Chester, Pennsylvania's housing projects in an official car borrowed from the health department. It was white, with blue and yellow stripes and lettering. It looked exactly like a police car.

"She didn't want to talk to us," Claire said. "Her sister was there, and neither of them wanted anything to do with anyone from the government. She wouldn't answer our questions at all."

Patiently and politely, the two began sorting through the woman's refrigerator, making conversation and asking about what she liked. She thawed slowly, and then suddenly opened up, chatting about where she shopped and offering her WIC card so they could check the government's records of what she had bought.

By the third day, clues began to emerge. There were a few foods that all the patients ate: 2 percent milk, American cheese. There were a few foods that none of them had eaten, things that had transmitted listeria in past outbreaks: no soft cheeses like Brie or queso fresco, and no pate. And there was one food that seemed to stand out.

"We were at one patient's house, and she mentioned the things that she and her husband liked: pot roast, pastrami, hot dogs," Sami said. "But when we went to the refrigerator, all we saw was turkey: turkey pastrami, turkey hot dogs. And when we asked her about it, she said, oh, she forgot to mention it, but her husband had a heart condition, and they were trying to eat more healthfully. So everything they once ate that was made out of beef or pork, they bought the turkey version now."

They compared their records. At every single household they had visited, there had been some turkey product in the refrigerator—turkey bacon, ground turkey, sliced turkey breast. The investigators had their hypothesis.

———

More precision was needed, to define what had caused the outbreak and to find the contaminated food in time to shut the outbreak down. The team devised a study, a much more detailed questionnaire that asked about symptoms, travel, past medical history, and eating habits. It was eighteen pages long and included seventy-five different types of food; for each one, participants had to choose whether they ate the food almost every day, three to four times a week, once or twice a week, once or twice a month, or never. It asked about turkey items, and also about cheese (block, sliced, shredded, and singly wrapped slices), lettuce (heads and prewashed bags), five types of milk, two kinds of hot dogs, two kinds of sausages, five kinds of lunch meat, and fresh, smoked, and frozen fish. It asked people to remember the brand names they bought, the restaurants they ate in, and the grocery stores where they shopped.

The study would be given to two groups of people: the patients who were part of the listeria outbreak, and controls who were not part of the outbreak, but were otherwise as much like the patients as possible. Case-control studies were a challenge for listeria investigations; because cases were rare and sporadic, it was easy to go wrong picking the matching controls, distorting the results. The team decided to pick as controls the listeriosis patients whose PFGE results did not match the outbreak strain. They had one essential thing in common with the cases—they had consumed some food that gave them listeria—and yet they were incontrovertibly not part of the outbreak.

There were plenty of controls to choose from: By September 10, the CDC lab had gotten isolates from fifty-six patients, but found only twelve among them whose PFGE pattern matched the outbreak strain. The rest were random, sporadic cases infected with a slightly different strain of the bacteria, a demonstration of the difficulty of lifting the signal of an outbreak out of the surrounding noise.

The thirty-minute questionnaire was designed to be given over the phone by employees of the state health departments. On September 12, Claire and Sami faxed the questionnaires to the states and got ready to hold questioner training sessions over the phone. That week, the outbreak picked up speed. There were twenty-six confirmed cases nationally, in Pennsylvania, Maryland, Connecticut, Michigan, and New York state. Four people were known to have died.

The study results came in quickly: names of groceries, names of restaurants, and a huge matrix of brand names, food types, and frequencies. It was more than the team, with their limited laptop power, could make sense of. On September 20, Sami bundled up the first thirty-eight responses, nineteen patients and nineteen controls, and took them back to Atlanta, to work with a senior statistician named Mike Hoekstra. Claire was not available—she was on her way to a wedding in Chicago—and Sami had a powerful reason for making the trip. Scott had been in the Philippines since August 9, and they had barely been able to speak; CDC rules limited employees on overseas assignment to one six-minute personal phone call every seven days. Now he was back in Atlanta, but only briefly. His supervisors were sending him to rural Africa the next week.

Sami and Hoekstra worked through the weekend, breaking for a few hours late Saturday night so Sami could go home to Scott. By Sunday evening, they had an answer. Out of the seventy-five different food items on the questionnaire, one was strongly associated with the patients' illness. It was one of the most common foods in the diet of an American trying to be healthy: turkey breast sliced in a deli.

———

As a culprit for the outbreak, though, "turkey breast" was still not good enough. The team needed a brand and a type, and there seemed to be dozens: smoked, herbed, low-salt, Cajun, whole-breast, chopped-pressed-formed, with sugar and without. Most of the participants could say which type they preferred, though not all. Some, so ill they could not speak for themselves, were represented in the study by family members who had limited information about their preferences.

Patients had difficulty remembering what brand of turkey they purchased, but they could almost always remember where they shopped. That provided the next clue. The team recruited fresh staff from state health departments, and from the U.S. Department of Agriculture, which had joined the investigation, and sent them into every establishment mentioned in a case-patient's study responses: fifty-seven delis, free-standing and inside supermarkets, in seven states. The searchers checked labels in deli cases, refrigerators, and storage freezers, and paged through stacks of invoices, multipage sheafs of carbons that stores received several times a week.

"We found out pretty quickly that brand names don't tell you much, because a single plant belonging to a single company could produce multiple brands of turkey," Claire said. "But we found out from USDA that there were these things called establishment numbers that were unique identifiers for each plant and that had to be on every product. So we also collected those."

The result was another welter of information. Some of the groceries carried thirty different types of turkey. The team gathered all the establishment numbers, matched them to the patients, ranked them by the frequency with which they appeared, and gave them to the USDA. The agency began looking at the list, planning its side of the investigation. And then a finding came from left field that cut them all off.

New York City, it turned out, had its own program of deli inspection, run by the New York state Department of Agriculture and Markets. On September 3, an inspector on a routine visit to a deli in Manhattan had opened a heat-sealed package of turkey breast, sliced some of the meat on the deli's slicer, and taken it back as a lab sample. The state's agriculture lab had performed the usual tests on the sample. It contained listeria. Then the lab had run PFGE on the listeria. It matched the outbreak strain.

It was a clue—perhaps. The slicer could have contaminated the turkey. There was no packaging left to say where the meat had come from; the deli owner had discarded the wrapper after the inspector's visit. The owner could not remember what brand he had bought, but the records of the distributor he ordered from provided an answer. It was a brand made by a single source: a plant in Franconia, Pennsylvania, outside Philadelphia, that belonged to Wampler Foods Inc. It was a subsidiary of Pilgrim's Pride Corp. of Texas, the second largest poultry company in the United States.

Over the next two days, Sami and Claire finished looking at the list of establishment numbers. One establishment showed up more than any of the others. It was the Wampler plant. In the first week of October, investigators from the CDC and the USDA's Food Safety and Inspection Service went into the plant. Claire and Sami went with them.

The outbreak had grown to forty cases, in seven states. Seven of the patients had died, and three had miscarried.

————

The Philadelphia health department lies just six blocks from the elegant townhouses of Rittenhouse Square; from the front door, you can look directly up Broad Street, the north-south spine of the central city, to the elegant City Hall topped by the benignly brooding statue of founder William Penn. But on the block the department stands on, gentrification has not yet arrived. It is a low building of glass block and blue-green glazed tile, wedged between two parking lots fenced with chain-link.

The department had given the team an upstairs conference room. They shoved its battered wood tables together into working areas: one for the constantly humming fax machines spitting out questionnaires from the different state departments, and one for the computers where Nicole Baker and veterinary student Suzanne Young, who had replaced Michelle Jefferson, typed in the questionnaire responses. There were stacks of blank questionnaires and other stacks of completed ones. There were Post-its and lists of telephone numbers tacked to the walls, and several dozen empty Diet Coke cans.

"The shoe-leather detective work, that's the part of the EIS that people think about," Sami said. "But the hardest part comes when you have to sit in front of the computer and enter your data and try to be extremely methodical and precise, so you can get to the bottom of the outbreak with certainty."

The team had gathered data on more than 150 different listeriosis patients who were newly diagnosed, hospitalized with sepsis and meningitis or at home recovering, or dead. They were unlikely to all be members of the outbreak, but the PFGE for many of them had not yet been completed. And if they were not outbreak patients, they were eligible to be controls for the study, so it was important to keep track of them all.

Each day, there were phone conversations with the foodborne supervisors in Atlanta and with the lab. State departments would call with information on new patients and questions about lab results, or because their interviewers were having difficulties with the study questionnaire. The USDA side of the investigation was continuing also: Every day or two, there were conference calls involving the team, the CDC, the state departments, the Food Safety and Inspection Service and the USDA's labs. Some days, there were more than twenty people on the line. The calls took hours.

"I felt like I was back in the ICU," Sami said. "You have a patient in front of you who's extremely sick, who could die, and you're going to stay at that person's bedside all night, doing whatever you can to keep them alive. I felt the same kind of urgency in this outbreak—but the patients we were trying to save, we couldn't see. And we knew there were plenty of others out there at risk."

It was a group of only women. They had been working in close proximity, for at least sixteen hours a day, for six weeks. On a day in

October, Nicole looked up from her computer and asked if anyone could spare a tampon. Sami, who had been feeling sick since she toured the turkey plant, looked up, too.

"You guys are having your periods?" she asked. "That's weird. I haven't had mine."

It took a moment for that to sink in.

Claire got up. She had been too busy to meet most of the Philadelphia department, but she was still interested in sexually transmitted diseases, and she had made friends in the STD clinic downstairs. She ran downstairs, and came back with two pregnancy tests. She handed them to Sami.

Sami headed for the bathroom. A few minutes later, she was back, holding one stick-like test in front of her. In the two tiny windows on its surface, there were two parallel pink lines.

"Is this positive?" she asked.

Claire examined it. She had worked in a molecular biology lab after college. "I'm pretty sure that's positive," she said.

Nicole and Suzanne applauded. Sami shook her head. "I don't think it's positive," she said. "I'm going to try again."

A few minutes later, she was back again. The second test looked like the first one: two windows, two thick parallel lines. Sami looked stunned. "It's positive," she said.

The other three whooped and hugged her. They chattered about how long it would take to tell Scott in Africa. Through her shock, Sami barely heard them. She and Scott wanted children and had planned to try before the first EIS year was over. She had not expected they would succeed quite so soon.

The women's excitement faded as they realized the situation's complexities. Sami was pregnant—and she was leading an investigation of a pathogen that attacked pregnant women and caused them to miscarry. And she was, in addition, stressed, sleep-deprived, and in the poorest nutritional shape since her residency.

On the way back to the hotel, after midnight, Claire bought her some prenatal vitamins.

The investigators had two avenues open to them. They could check the plant's environment for current colonies of listeria, looking in the cold, damp places that the bacteria preferred. And they could check the food the plant produced, to see whether listeria had been present in the past few months. By regulation, food processors kept "shelf-life" samples of every production run, sealed and chilled in storage. It made a kind of archive that could be referred back to if anything went wrong.

The plant was not a slaughterhouse. Turkeys were killed by a supplier, and arrived at the plant as carved-up carcasses to be turned into processed meat. The investigators toured it thoroughly, swabbing the environment at fifty-seven different spots and sending the swabs for analysis. They also took ten shelf-life samples from the archive, and seven samples from meat that was being produced at the time.

One of the shelf-life samples was a package of turkey pastrami. When it was opened and tested, it yielded listeria—not the outbreak strain, but a new strain. In response, Wampler launched a voluntary recall of 295,000 pounds of turkey and turkey pastrami that had been produced on the same day as the shelf-life sample.

There was still no culprit food, and the search for it was about to become more complicated. New York's agriculture department had returned to the Manhattan deli to get more information from its owner. In their second interview, he admitted that he might also have bought some turkey from a jobber, a man who had a small business buying meat and reselling it. That turkey came from a different plant: JL Foods Inc. of Camden, New Jersey, thirty miles from the Wampler plant. Two days later, analysis of a turkey breast sample from a Harlem deli, one that had been visited while the investigators were tracing patients' purchases, found the outbreak strain of listeria as well. But the deli's records were incomplete. It could have come from Wampler, or from JL Foods, or from one of two other plants as well.

The USDA began investigating the other three plants. On October 11, their attention was drawn back to Wampler: twenty-five of the fifty-seven environmental samples contained listeria. The next day, the PulseNet lab yielded the PFGE analysis: Two swabs taken from floor drains contained the outbreak strain. Wampler widened its recall to

27.4 million pounds of turkey, everything its plant had produced between May 1 and October 11. It closed its plant for cleaning, temporarily laying off 750 employees.

———

On October 25, the CDC's hotline received a phone call. It concerned a plumber in Massachusetts. He had been very ill. He had listeriosis, he was infected with the outbreak strain, and he had a story to tell.

The plumber was a healthy young man who usually made his own lunches. On October 5, a Saturday, he had bought some sliced turkey at a local market. He had eaten some that day, and some the next, and on Monday morning had made himself a sandwich and put it in his cooler to take to work. Sometime before lunch, though, he felt so sick that he drove himself to the emergency room. He had been hospitalized for almost a week. The sandwich had remained in his cooler.

With the help of his girlfriend, the Massachusetts health department had retrieved the sandwich and sent it to their public health lab for analysis. It contained the outbreak strain. The man's girlfriend had retrieved the wrapping from the turkey and called the market where he bought it, reading them the codes from the printed label stuck to the white deli paper. The market staff thought it was the turkey that had just been recalled—turkey produced by Wampler Foods.

USDA investigators descended on the market to double-check its records and inventory. It had bought turkey from Wampler, they discovered, but it had bought turkey from JL Foods as well.

On October 29, at a "listeria summit" in Washington, D.C., the new chief of the USDA's Food Safety and Inspection Service criticized the current meat inspection system. "Your system is broken, and it needs to be repaired," Gary McKee told a gathering of meat producers.

Two days later, as the outbreak cases rose to fifty, the USDA's lab also found the outbreak strain of bacteria in food samples. It was in a never-opened package of turkey breast, made by JL Foods, that the USDA had found in a store in Pennsylvania. The strain was also in an already opened package of turkey that had been retrieved from a deli in Harlem where one of the case-patients had shopped. For the past six months, according to the deli owner's records, the store had bought turkey from only one place: JL Foods. The New Jersey company, a family-owned concern with 150 employees, recalled 200,000 pounds of turkey meat and closed up shop to be cleaned.

By mid-November, the outbreak appeared to be ending. The USDA reported the results of its inspections. It found no listeria in the two other plants the Manhattan deli had named as possibilities. It found one listeria isolate, not the outbreak strain, on a forklift in the JL Foods plant. And it also found listeria—again, not the outbreak strain—in one of the 100 samples submitted by Wampler from the tons of turkey the company had recalled. On November 13, the USDA allowed the Wampler plant to open again. One day later, the agency allowed the JL Foods plant to reopen as well.

Six days after that, the USDA found one more sample of listeria, in another unopened retail package of turkey that had originated at JL Foods. The company recalled another 4.2 million pounds of turkey. Because the closure and cleaning had come after that sample was collected, the USDA did not force the plant to close again.

Overall, more than 32 million pounds of turkey were recalled during the outbreak. It was the second-largest meat recall in U.S. history. The final case count was fifty-four, with three miscarriages and eight deaths.

———

The last outbreak-related case of listeria, confirmed by PFGE, was discovered November 27. The investigators waited tensely through one incubation period before concluding that cases had come to an end. By Christmas, they were ready to declare the outbreak over.

They could never say with certainty if one company was the source of the outbreak. It was possible that both plants had been contaminated by some third party; the USDA, noticing that only thirty miles separated the two, had begun an investigation into any suppliers they had in common.

To the CDC team, though, the question of source was irrelevant. It was possible the listeria had been carried in from the outside; because the bug lives freely in the environment, it was also possible that it had floated in on its own. The issue was rather that, once inside the plants, the bug had not been completely controlled. The turkey had been cooked, and the cooking would have killed any listeria in the raw meat. The contamination must have occurred somewhere between cooking and packaging, though the USDA had not pinpointed where.

"We're confident that our investigation correctly led us to both plants, because the outbreak strain was in the environment of the first one and in the food products of the second," Sami said. "We can't say which is the primary one to blame, but blame isn't the issue; we're not trying to blame anyone, we're just trying to protect the public. And both plants did the right thing by recalling their product—which was agonizing for them, because it's a huge financial loss."

After Epi-Aids end, the team members write a memo for the record, giving a narrative of the investigation and explaining their conclusions and their proofs. When Claire and Sami assembled all their data to prepare the memo, they discovered something interesting: The three babies, the ones whose cases had sounded the alarm, were not part of the outbreak. Their PFGE patterns had not matched the outbreak strain.

"It's bizarre," Claire said. "They were the reason that we sounded the alarm, that gave us a chance to start looking around and asking whether there were other cases out there. And yet they were totally a red herring, not part of the outbreak at all."

SIX

AIDS

1981, Los Angeles

Los Angeles was just about the last place Wayne X. Shandera wanted to end up.

The wiry-haired physician had gone to college at Rice University in Houston, crossed the country to medical school at Johns Hopkins University in Baltimore, and then crossed back for residency at Stanford University outside San Francisco. Now he was wondering whether to pack up again. He had been admitted to the Epidemic Intelligence Service, and the group had asked him to list his preferences for an assignment.

Shandera was twenty-nine years old, a devout Catholic who read three languages and was an accomplished organist. He loved living in the Bay Area; he liked the climate and the architecture, and he felt at home in the left-leaning intellectual discourse that simmered in its bookstores and coffee shops. Shandera had moved to San Francisco in 1977, the year that activist Harvey Milk was elected to the city's board of supervisors. Milk was the first openly gay man to win a popular

99

election anywhere in America. When he was murdered a year later, gay men poured into the city, transforming its colorful, casual decadence into a nexus of sexual flamboyance and political fury. But Shandera had little contact with gay San Francisco. Heterosexual, socially conservative, and somewhat shy, he would rather have gone to a chamber music concert than a Pride parade.

At the moment, he was unsure where to go. Conventional CDC wisdom held that headquarters offered the best EIS assignments. Atlanta made personal sense as well. Shandera's father was ill with colon cancer in San Antonio, and he had left the promising beginnings of a relationship in Baltimore three years before. In Atlanta, he thought, he would have easy airplane access in both directions. On the other hand, he had just finished three years of caring for patients. He had not had a course in statistics or epidemiology since his second year of medical school, and he was weak in the necessary skills of sleuthing out the details of outbreaks and writing coherent narratives about them. He might, he thought, get more practice in a city or state health department.

EIS matching lets candidates list up to ten choices. Shandera studied the list of possible postings, and put the Louisiana health department first, followed by eight jobs in Atlanta, and the Los Angeles County health department dead last. It was a low probability, he thought; the matchers never worked their way that far down a candidate's list.

In June 1980, the notice arrived: After training in Atlanta, Shandera was to pack up his Stanford apartment and move south to Los Angeles.

He was horrified. His colleagues were dismissive.

"You're not going to find anything to work on there," his cardiology professor said. "Except for a bunch of sexually transmitted diseases."

He had no idea how prophetic a statement that was.

———

It looked, at first, as though Shandera's derisive professor had been wrong. There were plenty of diseases in Los Angeles. There was a cluster of miscarriages in Long Beach; two outbreaks of diarrhea, one in a day care center and one spread throughout the city; a set of hepatitis cases among women who donated their blood plasma; and a puzzling outbreak of epidemic neuromyasthenia, a syndrome of headache, fever, and muscle weakness, among patients of a neurologist in Pacific Palisades.

He did not solve all of the outbreaks, though they kept him busy. He worked hard, but he was unhappy. Nothing he was doing seemed novel, and he had been attracted to the EIS by the hope that he could help identify new health problems. Twice in the past five years, the group's members had helped identify previously unrecognized diseases. In the summer of 1976, they had scrambled to an epidemic of pneumonia that sickened 221 people and killed thirty-four at an American Legion convention in a hotel in Philadelphia; by the end of the year, CDC scientists had identified the pathogen causing it, dubbed the illness Legionnaires' disease, and exposed it as the cause of two other, never-solved outbreaks in 1965 and 1968. Two months before Shandera joined the EIS, in May 1980, the CDC had linked fifty-five severe cases of fever, rash, and Group A *Streptococcus* infection, a constellation of symptoms dubbed toxic shock syndrome, to women's use of high-absorbency tampons. Nothing that he was seeing in Los Angeles promised the excitement of those discoveries.

He worried, too, that he wasn't learning enough epidemiology. He missed the intense supervision of residency. Most of his colleagues at the county health department had master's degrees in public health. He felt they were all on the same level; it made it hard to find a mentor. He had chosen public health, to start with, out of a sense that he wanted to make more of a difference than he would working one-to-one with patients in a hospital. In Los Angeles, he couldn't see any evidence that he was making much of a difference at all.

The clincher was that he loathed Los Angeles. In San Francisco, he had biked everywhere; now he owned an old Mustang and was immersed every day in the city's desperate traffic. The air quality was very bad that year—"Some days we couldn't see across the street," said Frank Sorvillo, an epidemiologist who shared a cubicle with him—and the frank materialism of the city grated on Shandera's sensibilities.

"In one day, I would see twenty migrant workers living in a garage in East Los Angeles, and then have to drive through Bel Air, and be staggered by the contrasts," he said. "It was disturbing, and hard to work in. I was at odds with the city most of the time."

In the spring, when EIS slots opened up for the incoming class, Shandera asked the corps to transfer him. They offered him a job working for Dr. Paul Blake in the enteric diseases branch in Atlanta, starting in late July 1981. He accepted.

———

In addition to the outbreaks that Shandera worked on, there was something else percolating through southern California that spring. Some of the health department's epidemiologists heard reports from doctors they knew, that patients in practices in the San Fernando Valley were complaining of swollen lymph nodes and stubborn low-grade fevers. There was no obvious diagnosis. Those symptoms could signal the start of lymphoma, a cancer of the immune system that attacked a particular type of white blood cell, but tests were finding no trace of cancer. Most of the patients, the doctors said, were men.

At about the same time, a pathologist at University of Southern California called Sorvillo. He had evidence of cancers in a cluster of six male patients. But there was something odd about what he was seeing through the microscope; the pathology of these lymphomas was like nothing he had seen before. One of the patients was still in the hospital, and Shandera and Sorvillo went to interview him. The man was a drug addict, but there was nothing else extraordinary about him, nothing that would predispose him to an unusual lymphatic cancer. They let the case go.

At University of California-Los Angeles, anomalous cases were showing up as well. They were finding their way to Dr. Michael S. Gottlieb, an assistant professor of immunology who had joined the medical school staff in the summer of 1980. Like Shandera, Gottlieb had come from Stanford, and they had known each other there slightly. Gottlieb, who was four years older, had been a Howard Hughes Institute research fellow on the immunology service when

Shandera had rotated through as a resident, and had gone over cases and journal articles with the younger doctor.

Gottlieb's specialty was the immunology of organ transplantation. At Stanford, he had looked for ways to persuade the body to accept transplants without using drugs to suppress the immune system, the only way known to keep the organs from being rejected as foreign. Unlike Shandera, Gottlieb liked Los Angeles. While at Stanford, he had spent some time at UCLA studying bone-marrow transplants, and the university had invited him to move south and open an immunologic research lab.

Gottlieb was one of two attending physicians—senior doctors who supervise the training of younger ones—on the immunology service of UCLA School of Medicine. On a slow day in March 1981, he asked Dr. Howard Schanker, a fellow working under him, to survey the hospital for patients whose cases might present teaching opportunities.

Gottlieb's office was in the hospital basement. Schanker left for the upper floors. Very shortly afterward, he was back.

"He had a quizzical look on his face," Gottlieb said. "He said, 'There is a guy upstairs whose infections are really kind of strange.'"

The man's name was Michael. He was thirty-three years old, tall and good-looking, with short, peroxided hair and prominent cheekbones. He was a model, he confided; he'd had his face enhanced with cheekbone implants.

He was also quite sick. He had been ill since October with a fluctuating fever and swollen glands in his neck and under his collarbone. The glands had gone down, but the fever would not go away. He had lost a lot of weight, and now he was losing his hair. He had raw patches of fluffy white growths—candidiasis, a yeast-like fungus, as well as herpes virus—inside his mouth, between his buttocks, and on his index fingers. The medical ward had run some tests already: He had an organism called cytomegalovirus in his urine, his white blood cell count was low, and one particular class of white cell, the T-lymphocytes, were much fewer than they ought to be. All the findings pointed to the same conclusion: His immune system was not working the way it should.

There was no indication, though, why that should be so. He had not had cancer or chemotherapy. He had not had an organ transplant. He was not elderly—aging wears down the immune system—and he did not have an inherited immune deficiency. Children born with that condition seldom survived long, and certainly not to Michael's age. There was no evidence that he had suffered any medical or environmental insults that would impair his immunity. His symptoms were treatable, but his underlying condition was unexplained.

When Gottlieb and Schanker arrived at his room, Michael was on the phone. He was telling a friend, archly, "These doctors tell me I am one sick queen."

Michael's symptoms were treated successfully, and he was discharged a week later. A month later, he was readmitted to the hospital, still feverish but now almost unable to breathe. A resident who had treated him the first time, Dr. Robert Wolf, spotted him on the same ward. Knowing the man's immune system had been depressed before, and fearing a new infection had taken hold, Wolf ordered a chest X-ray and a bronchoscopy, a direct viewing of the airways through a flexible tube that lets its operator bring up specimens from deep in the lungs.

The results were perplexing and alarming. The air spaces in Michael's lungs were filled with millions of *Pneumocystis carinii,* a microscopic protozoan that attacked cancer patients and recipients of transplants, people whose immune systems had essentially ceased to function. Pneumocystis was so rare that Gottlieb, a specialist in transplant immunology, had never seen a case.

News of his case buzzed through the Los Angeles medical grapevine. Shortly after Michael had been readmitted in April, Gottlieb got a call from Dr. Peng Thim Fan, a rheumatologist, and Dr. Joel Weisman, an osteopath who had a general practice treating gay men. Weisman was also seeing patients with unexplained fevers and weight loss, lymphadenopathy, and cytomegalovirus infection. Gottlieb arranged to have two of the patients admitted to UCLA. By the time they arrived, they too had pneumonia. Before being put on respirators, they were bronchoscoped.

Like Michael, their lungs were full of pneumocystis, and their blood chemistries were awry. Their overall T-cell counts were not only low, but out of balance. There were almost no helper T-cells, the white blood cells that help manufacture antibodies to mount an immune defense against pathogens. There were far too many cytotoxic and suppressor T-cells, the ones that kill the invading organisms and then shut down the immune response.

All three men were seriously, inexplicably ill. Michael never left the hospital. He died May 3.

"In medicine," Gottlieb said, "one case of something is a curiosity. Two cases is very interesting. But a third case, that makes you ask: Is this going to be something big?"

Gottlieb thought the answer was yes. Weisman was seeing more patients with stubborn fevers and fungal infections, and another friend had told him of a fourth case of cytomegalovirus infection, in a hospital in another part of town. If the mystery syndrome was sprinkled throughout Los Angeles, surely it would be of concern elsewhere also. He called the *New England Journal of Medicine,* the most respected medical journal in the country.

"I said we had at least three cases, all gay men, all with pneumocystis pneumonia, all with severe immune deficiency—something was up," Gottlieb said. "I told them I thought it might be bigger than Legionnaires' disease."

The journal's editors were interested, but not enough to bend the journal's strict rules. It would take at least three months to get an article reviewed by other doctors, approved, and into print, they said. And while it was being approved, Gottlieb would not be able to publish anything else about the mystery syndrome: The journal had an ironclad policy of many years' standing that anything appearing in its pages could not show up in another journal first.

There was a compromise, the editor-in-chief suggested. If Gottlieb wanted to alert the medical world rapidly, he could consider placing an article in the Morbidity and Mortality Weekly Report, the weekly bulletin published by the CDC. The *New England Journal* did not consider the staple-bound newsletter, the size of a folded sheet of paper, to be any kind of competition. If Gottlieb's news appeared there first, he could still write a paper for the prestigious outlet later.

Gottlieb was a researcher and clinician; he had very little contact with the world of public health. But he did, he realized, know someone at the CDC. He called Wayne Shandera.

―――――

Shandera and Gottlieb had always planned to get together in Los Angeles, perhaps to work together on a project that combined their interests. Shandera had liked the idea, but the realities of health department work had gotten in the way. Here, though, was an opportunity to explore a truly interesting outbreak, even if it was occurring just as he planned to leave Los Angeles for good. EIS members were supposed to publish in the MMWR, as it was called, if possible. The half-sized booklet was the best-read magazine that no one had ever heard of; thousands of state health department epidemiologists and university infectious disease physicians read it every week.

So Shandera welcomed the call from his onetime attending, even though Gottlieb was carefully nonspecific.

"I said something like, 'Hi, Wayne, how are you, I'm sorry I haven't seen you lately—and, by the way, are you hearing anything at the health department about anything unusual among gay men?' " Gottlieb said. "Because I wondered whether someone else perhaps was already on to this. I can still remember him saying no, and feeling a bit let down. Because if no one else had noticed it, maybe we were overreacting."

Shandera promised to look around. He did not have to look far. One of the department's epidemiologists had gotten a report from St. John's Hospital in Santa Monica of a patient hospitalized with pneumocystis. He decided to investigate. As a health department employee, he was allowed access to otherwise private medical records. He drove down to Santa Monica.

The patient was a twenty-nine-year-old man. He, too, was very ill. He had had Hodgkin's disease, a lymphoma, three years earlier, but had recovered after radiation therapy. There was no evidence that the cancer had recurred, but he had had pneumocystis pneumonia for more than a month. Cytomegalovirus had been found in his system as well.

"He looked like the cancer patients I had seen at Stanford—like someone who had been through a lot of chemotherapy, or was suffering from very end-stage cancer," Shandera said. "He was lying in bed, wasted, looking very thin. Pneumocystis pneumonia causes air hunger; you develop cyanosis, purpling and mottling of the skin, and you lose all your peripheral fat, like a famine victim."

The man's lover was with him, in the waiting room of the intensive care unit. Shandera talked to both men, and then drove back to Los Angeles. Epidemiologically speaking, the patient was not exactly like the others, because he had something in his recent past—cancer and cancer treatment—that could have disrupted his immune system. Still, the pneumocystis and cytomegalovirus were unusual enough to be striking. Shandera called Gottlieb back.

"There's another case," he said, adding almost as an afterthought: "This one is homosexual too."

Gottlieb felt the hair on the back of his neck bristle. "I knew it had to be related," he said. "We had to get this out."

Shandera's predecessor at L.A. County had lived in Beverly Hills, but Shandera had chosen instead to live in West Los Angeles, a raffish, not-yet-renovated mix of artists and ethnicities. His landlords were Armenian. A librarian for UCLA was upstairs. The program director for the major public radio station lived across the street.

On a blistering Sunday afternoon in mid-May, the two doctors met at Shandera's apartment. Gottlieb brought the medical charts of the three patients he had seen and the fourth who had been sent to him. Shandera had the paperwork on the cancer patient in Santa Monica, who had died shortly after Shandera interviewed him.

Riffling through the pages of treatment histories and test results, they drafted a short paper, only nine paragraphs long. It began matter-of-factly:

> In the period October 1980–May 1981, 5 young men, all active homosexuals, were treated for biopsy-confirmed *Pneu-*

mocystis carinii pneumonia at 3 different hospitals in Los Angeles, California. Two of the patients died. All 5 patients had laboratory-confirmed previous or current cytomegalovirus infection and candidal mucosal infection.

The two doctors followed with a description of all five patients: Patient 1, thirty-three years old, diagnosed with pneumonia in March after two months of fever and liver dysfunction; dead. Patient 2, thirty years old, diagnosed with pneumonia in April after five months of fever and liver dysfunction, still experiencing daily fevers even though the pneumonia was gone. Patient 3, thirty, hospitalized in February with pneumonia. Patient 4, twenty-nine, successfully treated for Hodgkin's disease three years ago, diagnosed with pneumonia in February; dead. Patient 5, thirty-six, diagnosed with widespread yeast infection in September, hospitalized with pneumonia in April, still suffering from candida despite repeated courses of drugs.

There were no obvious reasons, the doctors added, why this should be an outbreak. The patients had very little in common.

> The patients did not know each other and had no known common contacts. . . . The 5 did not have comparable histories of sexually transmitted disease. . . . Two of the 5 reported having frequent homosexual contacts with various partners. All 5 reported using inhalant drugs, and 1 reported parenteral drug abuse. Three patients had profoundly depressed numbers of thymus-dependent lymphocyte cells.

And in a foray into preliminary analysis, Gottlieb and Shandera underlined how odd these occurrences were.

> The occurrence of pneumocystis in these 5 previously healthy individuals without a clinically apparent underlying immunodeficiency is unusual. The fact that these patients were all homosexuals suggests an association between some aspect of a homosexual lifestyle or disease acquired through sexual contact and Pneumocystis pneumonia in this population.

When the paper was done, the authors titled it, "Pneumocystis Pneumonia in Homosexual Men—Los Angeles." Gottlieb signed his name to it, along with the names of Schanker, Fan, Weisman, and two other doctors who had seen the five patients. Shandera did not sign his name. By CDC tradition, EIS officers who contributed to the MMWR did not get named credit on papers; he was listed only as an anonymous representative of the "Field Services Division, Epidemiology Program Office, CDC."

The next day, Shandera called the MMWR, and dictated the report over the phone. The transcribed text was passed up the line to Dr. James Curran, who was chief of the CDC's sexually transmitted diseases unit. He scrawled a note across the margins of the first page: "Hot stuff."

Despite that endorsement, the paper did not make it into the MMWR unchanged. When it ran, on June 5, 1981, its title had been edited down to "Pneumocystis pneumonia—Los Angeles." And it ran not on the cover of the booklet, but inside on pages two and three. The placement, and the words cut from the title, came from a combination of protectiveness, tact, and squeamishness. The report's staff were unsure how much attention should be drawn to a problem that appeared to be afflicting only homosexuals.

The following week, pursuing a tip, Shandera visited the intensive care unit at Los Angeles County Hospital. There were three men in the unit, all on respirators and dying. All three had pneumocystis pneumonia.

"That's when I knew that this was bigger than we realized," he said. "I thought, if you can find patients this easily, immediately after a published report of something that looked rare, then this outbreak is of major importance."

———

The disease that Gottlieb and Shandera described in their article was dubbed Acquired Immune Deficiency Syndrome—AIDS—in July 1982. The organism that causes it, human immunodeficiency virus, was recognized in 1983. By the end of 2003, almost 200,000 medical journal articles had been written on aspects of HIV infection and AIDS. Gottlieb and Shandera's was the first.

By the beginning of 2004, there had been more than 20 million deaths from AIDS across the globe. The estimated number of people living with HIV infection is more than 40 million.

Gottlieb, who was just beginning his medical career in 1981, spent it working on AIDS. As its editor had promised, the *New England Journal of Medicine* accepted his article on the first patients; its publication in December 1981 marked the first clinical description of the new syndrome in a major medical journal. He treated many of the disease's early victims in Los Angeles, including the movie star Rock Hudson. When Gottleib announced to a July 1985 press conference that Hudson was dying of AIDS, he forced the epidemic into the consciousness of mainstream America. He never went back to the transplant-immunity work for which UCLA had recruited him, and after eight years there did not receive tenure. Instead, he went into private practice and continued to do research.

Shandera took a quite different path. As he had planned, he left Los Angeles in July 1981, less than a month after the seminal paper was published. It was a tumultuous time for him. He had hoped reassignment to Atlanta would make it easier to see his ailing father in San Antonio; his father died in August. The potential relationship he planned to investigate in Baltimore did not materialize; they remained friends. He completed his second year in EIS in Atlanta. Several times, he dropped in on meetings of the CDC's early response to AIDS, a small task force of people pulled from specialties across the agency who were desperately trying to keep up with the rapidly emerging epidemic. Soon, though, the rigors of his new job pulled him away.

When his EIS stint ended, he left for a fellowship in clinical infectious disease research in Boston. He went into private practice in San Antonio, and then in Portland, and then returned to academic work in South Carolina, and then in Dallas, where he opened the first AIDS clinic in the city's largest public hospital.

"We had only two doctors, and at the time only one drug," he said. "We were on edge and emotional all the time. So many people were dying."

The institution, Parkland, was also a teaching hospital, and the experience there brought home to him that his greatest strength was his teaching skill. Afterward, he moved to Houston, where he joined the faculty of Baylor College of Medicine. He is an assistant professor—he never pursued tenure—and works weekly in the city's largest AIDS clinic. He supervises interns and residents, but much of his own research now is done on computers; he performs mathematical modeling of the potential further spread of AIDS. He reads German novels, does volunteer medical care in Central America, and visits his ninety-five-year-old mother, who still lives by herself in San Antonio.

He has wondered, sometimes, if leaving Los Angeles was the right decision. In that month between the paper's being published and his departing, he was surprised by the depth of his feelings for what seemed to be going on. In his last weeks, he pulled off a quick epidemiological study, talking his way into a gay community center in West Hollywood to ask men about the drugs they used, hoping to find a key to the disease's immune-system destruction. He found nothing of use.

He has never felt any ownership of the AIDS epidemic, or any sense that his name should be associated with it.

"If I hadn't been there, someone else would have reported these cases," he said. "If Mike hadn't written his paper, someone else would have written it. I happened to be there, and it fell to me to see the first cases, but I played such a bit part."

SEVEN

Uniformity

November–December 2002,
Atlanta

THE FIRST TIME THAT THE CLASS OF 2002 reassembled in Atlanta, it was a cool, sunny weekend morning in mid-autumn. The EIS class was massed in a hotel conference room two miles southeast of the CDC. The program's leadership had summoned them back from their assignments to undergo another new addition to the program: a basic officer training course.

They had had to dress up for it. All around the room, people whose concept of "uniform" was a matching set of surgical scrubs were tugging on the scratchy waistbands of wool regulation trousers. Men held grande lattes at arm's length, trying to keep the froth from landing on the plastic surface of mirror-shined lace-up shoes. Women craned their chins over their shoulders, fumbling with the brass buttons that held their floppy epaulets in place. Leigh Ramsey, an exercise physiologist who had become state officer for New Hampshire—a seven-time marathoner who usually wore denim skirts and little hooded sweat-shirts—was trying to cram her shoulder-length mane of curls under a dish-shaped military hat.

"I haven't done this since I was in kindergarten," she said, twisting the errant strands into an approximation of a braid and jamming the cap down over them in hopes they would stay put. "I don't think it's going to last very long."

A muted chatter rose from the seats around her. More than a third of the group had not seen each other since August. The night before, they had sat up late, talking and drinking. A few of them were frankly hungover, and most of the rest were muzzy-headed with fatigue.

Without warning, a bugle call cut through the babble. The group twisted in their chairs in sleep-tinged confusion: Why was someone playing something that sounded like a trumpet inside their hotel?

At the front of the room, a stocky man with brush-cut hair and a chest full of service ribbons pushed the off button on a tape recorder.

"That was the call to attention," said Commander Dana Taylor of the Commissioned Corps of the United States Public Health Service. "When you hear that, you should stop talking."

———

From its 1798 founding, the United States Public Health Service had kept watch over the health of the new United States by mounting guard over its then most important borders, the coasts and commercial waterways. Maritime commerce was not only one of the main drivers of the nascent economy; it was also one of the main routes by which infectious diseases could enter the new nation. The Marine Hospital Service, as it was first known, started out localized: Funding came from the government, but customs officials in the port cities supervised hospital administration and hiring. By the time the Civil War ended, Congress grew dissatisfied with local control and reorganized the service. It gave the group a chief—the supervising surgeon, later called the surgeon general—and created a military-style officer class of physicians, called the Commissioned Corps. Creating the Corps broke local control of the hospitals: Members were hired by the service, looked to the surgeon general as their commanding officer, and agreed to work wherever the surgeon general assigned them.

The service, renamed the Public Health Service in 1912, was the main federal health agency for 150 years. It had quarantine authority over vessels and immigrants, ruled over sanitation and sewage issues, and investigated epidemics. To help control outbreaks of disease, it launched the National Hygienic Laboratory, the first version of the National Institutes of Health, in 1887. By the twentieth century, though, its responsibilities shifted as states and cities founded their own public health departments. In 1953, it became part of the federal government's first cabinet-level health agency, the Department of Health, Education and Welfare, which was reorganized in 1979 into the Department of Health and Human Services.

In 2002, the Public Health Service still existed as a division of HHS, taking in 55,000 employees at the CDC, NIH, Agency for Toxic Substances and Disease Registry, Food and Drug Administration, Substance Abuse and Mental Health Services Administration, Agency for Healthcare Research and Quality, Health Resources and Services Administration, and Indian Health Service. The Commissioned Corps persisted also, with roughly 5,700 members—Ph.D.s, nurses, veterinarians, and dentists as well as doctors—scattered among the eight agencies. It had become one of seven uniformed services within the U.S. government, alongside the Army, Navy, Air Force, Marines, Coast Guard, and commissioned officers within the National Oceanic and Atmospheric Administration. It was led, technically at least, by the surgeon general, though most of its budget and personnel issues were handled by HHS's assistant secretary for health. At the CDC, there were about 300 corps members, roughly 10 percent of the agency's staff.

For physicians, joining the corps was the price of admission to the EIS; Ph.D.s, nurses, and other health professionals could choose whether or not to belong. There were powerful incentives, though. Corps members earned much better benefits than civilian HHS employees: Part of their pay was tax-free; their retirement plans were fully funded by the government; and they got thirty days of vacation per year, unlimited sick leave, free travel on military aircraft, and admission to the deeply discounted stores on military bases. In return, members wore a Navy-like uniform and swore the same commissioning oath given to members of the armed forces: "I will support and defend the Constitution of the United States against all enemies, foreign and domestic." The PHS added an extra clause to the oath: "I am willing to serve in any area or position or wherever the exigencies of the Service may require."

In practice, there was little downside to corps membership. Leaving could be costly: It took twenty years to be vested in the pension system, so officers who changed their minds and resigned their commissions faced starting their retirement savings from scratch. But the uniform was required only one day a week, and few veterans could remember anyone being sent to a post against their will. The Commissioned Corps had become a shadow personnel system within the federal health agencies, offering superior pay and easy promotions and transfers—extra rewards for which surprisingly little sacrifice was asked in return.

The 2001 anthrax attacks destroyed that comfortable status quo. The nationwide panic caused by the pathogen-loaded letters, which forced more than ten thousand people in four states onto antibiotics for sixty days, underlined that the country was vulnerable not just to deliberately caused disease outbreaks, but to epidemics of fear. The little-known Commissioned Corps was a ready-made homeland defense force, already committed by its oath to immediate action at the discretion of the surgeon general. The administration launched an effort to make the corps better organized and better known. That required reinforcing for its newest members just what they had committed themselves to.

Thus most of the 2002 class—minus foreign nationals who were ineligible for corps membership, and Ph.D.s and nurses who had opted not to join—found themselves in a suburban hotel, undergoing the first basic officer training course ever given to EIS members.

"We want to establish the flavor of a uniformed service that the corps is somewhat deficient in," said Taylor, who came from the staff of the Commissioned Officer Training Academy in Washington. "Our job is to instill in you as much pride and excitement in these uniforms as we can."

He sketched out their three-day lesson plan. They would study the history of the Public Health Service, the qualifications needed to join it, the rules for being promoted and going on leave, and the benefits they would accrue once they served, down to their right to a military funeral. They would learn to fill out corps paperwork, and there was a lot of paperwork. And they would cover military comportment: How to conduct a flag ceremony. How to stand at attention. How to discreetly eyeball the insignia on the other services' uniforms and know who outranked whom.

"Because we don't have our own installations, we depend on the other services for commissaries, PX, and the judge advocate general corps," Taylor said. "So we need to understand the practices that the other services use. You must pay respect; there are MPs out there just looking for work to do if you do not."

Taylor set the group to practicing salutes: stand at attention, bend the right arm and raise it to shoulder height, carefully cant the right hand so it was edge-on to the forehead, snap off a salute and return to attention again. He demonstrated. He showed them pictures: Keep the wrist straight; keep the fingers together; avoid palms turned outward like British paratroopers and pinkies tucked under like the Boy Scouts.

The practice did not go well. The class members saluted limply, with drooping elbows. They stood with their feet apart, forgetting the difference between "attention" and "at ease." Among the women, chignons came undone, sending their hair cascading over their collars.

Taylor looked dissatisfied. The class looked mutinous.

"You may think that you won't need this, " he said. "But even if you are just a lieutenant, you will. Lieutenant is a heavy rank. If I took you out on an aircraft carrier right now, ninety percent of the sailors on it would have to salute you."

———

Basic training ended after three days, but the uniforms continued to be a sore spot. To some of the class at least, they connoted a top-down hierarchy that felt at odds with public health's open, consultative style, and the classs members looked for ways to avoid wearing them.

To a degree, they had history on their side. For much of the EIS's history, the uniform-wearing part of Commissioned Corps membership had not been emphasized. Appearing in a military-style uniform with shiny shoes and a panel of service ribbons had been particularly uninteresting to the Vietnam-era enrollees who had chosen the CDC as an escape from military service. They had a jocular name for themselves—the "yellow berets"—and thirty years later, they made up a significant portion of the CDC's senior leadership.

Wednesday was uniform day. Wearing the uniform was technically mandatory, but in practice turned out to be only "strongly advised." The greater the distance from the CDC's headquarters building on Clifton Road, the less likely corps members were to wear it. In the satellite offices sprinkled around Atlanta, corps members put on the uniform if they liked not having to make wardrobe decisions that morning, or worked for a supervisor who required it, or needed to attend a meeting with senior staff who were sure to follow the rules and to scold those who did not. CDC staff assigned to state health departments preferred not to wear it, because it made them stand out so much from their local co-workers. Staff members working overseas were not compelled to wear it because they might be taken for American military officers, a mistake that could spur prejudice against their programs and in some countries would endanger their lives.

Even on the main campus, the embrace of the uniform was partial at best. Some took pride in the history it implied. Others worried that it was divisive, an unnecessary reminder that a corps member was getting better pay and benefits and easier promotions than an equally credentialed civil servant colleague one desk away.

The mix of attitudes gave the CDC, once a week, an odd piebald look. Four days out of five, the staff pouring into the Clifton Road buildings were indistinguishable from the researchers parking at Emory University's medical center next door: They wore jeans and Dockers, Tevas and ethnic jewelry, scientists' equivalent of a corporate dress code. On Wednesday, though, the crowds were sprinkled with the khaki and salt and pepper of corps uniforms. It made the agency look as though it had been infiltrated by military advisers overnight.

Permissiveness about the uniform ended almost exactly as the class of 2002 arrived. Part of that was a by-product of general post-9/11 tension. Some of the change, though, was due to a near-simultaneous government hire: On July 23, Dr. Richard Carmona had become the first surgeon general chosen by the Bush administration.

Carmona was a one-man health care system. He had been, in turn, a combat medic, nurse, trauma surgeon and hospital-system administrator in Arizona, as well as a deputy sheriff and SWAT team member. Before all that, though, he had been a high-school dropout from Spanish Harlem whose life was transformed when he enlisted in the Army. He had ended up as a Green Beret. In his worldview, military discipline, uniforms included, was an unconditionally positive thing. When he had been in office a few months, rumors began circulating that he planned to order the Commissioned Corps to wear its uniforms every day, and might ask the group to meet physical-fitness requirements as well.

In mid-November, Carmona made his first official visit to the CDC. A mandatory all-hands meeting was called; staff who could not fit into the main auditorium were told to watch his speech on live videocast. A superbly fit man with a relaxed manner, he came off as genial and even humble, joking about being caught eating fast food and urging staff members to contact him with ideas for emphasizing fitness and obesity prevention.

Carmona had on his PHS attire, the heavily braided vice-admiral's uniform that a surgeon general usually wears in public. He was piped into the auditorium and preceded by a color guard and a choir that sang the PHS anthem: "The mission of our service / Is known the world around; / In research and in treatment, / No equal can be found. / In the silent war against disease, / No truce is ever seen. / We serve on the land and the sea for humanity, / The Public Health Service team."

When he took questions, an audience member asked his plans for the Commissioned Corps.

"We have to increase our visibility," he said. "Much of the work that is done by the PHS is done anonymously. The public needs to know who we are."

After the speech, the 2002 class's discomfort over the uniforms increased. For a few of them, it sharpened into revolt. They talked about resigning their commissions, but hesitated: Most of them had chosen the EIS because they wanted to keep working for the CDC afterward, and they suspected quitting the corps would not look good on their records. Still they felt tricked, as though they had applied to enter the Peace Corps and found themselves hired into the infantry—though their situation was more analogous to someone who enrolled in the reserves planning only to be a weekend warrior, and unexpectedly found himself called to an actual war instead.

"I hate the whole uniform thing," one of the female physicians in the class said in a headquarters hallway one morning. "I feel like I'm playing dress-up when I wear it."

A few weeks earlier, to be ready for Carmona's appearance, she had ordered a few uniform pieces she was missing. The store where the orders were delivered was on an Air Force base northwest of Atlanta. When she drove in, a gate guard had saluted her car.

"I wanted to say to him, 'No, you don't understand, I should be saluting you,'" she said. "I couldn't do it because it would just get him in trouble and he wouldn't understand. But it is so wrong that I outrank him because I went to medical school. It's disrespectful to people who have committed their lives to the military, and it's not what I'm here for."

―――――

The emphasis on correct uniform-wearing seemed a distraction when there were more serious things to think about. The West Nile epidemic had subsided at last, but a troubling series of explosive stomach illnesses had begun cropping up on cruise ships. And members of the class had been recruited into a prevention campaign that was keeping some of them awake late at night, either working in their offices or fighting off nightmarish imaginings. They were working on smallpox.

Preparations for the possibility that smallpox could be used as a weapon against the United States had begun at the CDC almost immediately after the 2001 terrorist attacks, and intensified when the anthrax letters demonstrated how easily a bioterror agent could be disseminated. Before the end of 2001, the agency had launched training sessions for state health department employees and local first-responders, multiday courses that began with how to tell smallpox from other rash diseases, moved on to strategies for organizing vaccination campaigns once an attack had been detected, and finished by floating the uglier possibilities of an attack: calling in the National Guard to block off highways, for instance, or quelling citizens who were rioting to demand vaccine.

More than two hundred of the CDC's own staff, along with several hundred other public health workers, had passed through the sobering course. It often became contentious. Its basic assumption was that no one would be vaccinated until a case was detected. After that, vaccine would be distributed in a pattern that resembled the rings on a bull's-eye—first the household and medical contacts of the initial cases, then law enforcement and public health personnel dealing with the investigation, and then the contacts of all of those contacts. The plan was theoretically feasible, because smallpox vaccination could protect against developing the disease up to three days after someone was exposed to the virus. Nevertheless, it would not work, state and city workers told the CDC bluntly. Unless police and EMTs knew in advance that they were protected against the virus, there was no guarantee they would show up when a case was detected.

Throughout 2002, calls to change the plan and allow Americans to be vaccinated as a defense against any possible attack had been growing. The response at first had been simple: There was not enough vaccine to go around; only 15 million doses that dated back to the days before eradication remained in the federal stockpile. Shortly that argument became moot, as the government contracted for enough new vaccine to protect the entire country, and researchers discovered the old vaccine could be diluted 5-to-1 and remain potent. The new abundance immediately posed a new question: If more people than those immediately in danger could be vaccinated, then who should be?

It was not an easy question to answer, because it was not a benign vaccine. In those who had never been vaccinated before, it could cause life-threatening medical problems, and occasionally death, as well as many mild reactions that were nevertheless alarming. Rates of vaccine reactions were the main reason that U.S. vaccination had stopped when it did, eight years before smallpox was eradicated. Up to 130 million Americans, including a good proportion of the CDC's staff, had not been born when vaccination ceased, leaving them vulnerable to full-strength reactions. And because the vaccinia virus used in the vaccine was live and could spread from the vaccinated person to close contacts, the potential dangers of the vaccine were not limited to those who received it. Unvaccinated children, elderly and immunocompromised persons—of whom there were many more in 2002 than in the 1970s—would also be at risk.

Since the summer, federal health authorities had been arguing—mostly behind closed doors, but to a surprising degree in public—over balancing the risks of vaccination against the need to prepare for bioterrorism. Medical journal articles offered dueling models of how fast a smallpox epidemic would spread. Polls reported that Americans were willing to volunteer for the vaccination because they felt so at risk. In mid-December, President George W. Bush ended the suspense, announcing that 500,000 members of the military and about 450,000 public health and health care workers would receive the shot, but discouraging average citizens from seeking it. (As military commander-in-chief, he would be vaccinated, he said, but his wife and daughters would not.)

The announcement did little to diminish the EIS class's tension over smallpox. Some of their CDC co-workers had already been vaccinated: not only the poxvirus scientists, who handled the secret smallpox stockpile and were vaccinated every year, but staff epidemiologists and second-year EIS officers who had volunteered to be on the CDC's new smallpox rapid-response teams. No one had yet asked the 2002 class to be vaccinated, but they had begun receiving emails asking, if they were offered the vaccine, would they take it.

"I said yes," said Kirsten Ernst, the nurse who led the Mississippi West Nile deployment. She had been recruited into the smallpox effort on a thirty-day loan from her regular job at the Agency for Toxic

Substances and Disease Registry, a CDC division that dealt with environmental contamination.

"They asked, do you have young children, or are you or your significant other pregnant or trying to get pregnant, or nursing," she said. "And I don't fall into any of those categories right now, so it seems better to take it now. If something were to happen, we're deployable. We're the front line, when it comes to health care. So I think we need to prepare, not just education-wise, but healthwise."

A number of her classmates had also been yanked from their jobs to join the smallpox effort, serving thirty- or sixty-day stints preparing education materials or manning hotlines that provided information to physicians. About two-thirds of the class had escaped the duty so far, but it had not kept them from thinking about smallpox. A lot of the CDC seemed to be thinking about the disease; concern about it hung in the air like a barely audible, discordant hum. The EIS members remembered their summer training: They would be the first responders if a smallpox attack ever came.

"Smallpox is our doomsday scenario," said Doug Hamilton, the chief of the EIS. "If we ever get into a situation where it appears that smallpox has been released, we're going to call everybody."

———

Kirsten was one of those who had no difficulties with the uniform. She often wore it on days when it was not required. She preferred the informal khaki skirt and short-sleeved blouse, and had mastered the knack of sweeping her shoulder-length blonde hair into a smooth twist that anchored her cap. As a nurse, she had not been required to join the Commissioned Corps. She had chosen it.

"I wore a uniform as a nurse, so that wasn't an issue," she said. "And I did a lot of research before I chose, so I knew what was expected. I think, after September 11, it's more important for the Public Health Service to be visible. And members of the public have asked me about it, when they see me out on the street. I think they like knowing we exist."

Research scientists were also allowed to choose whether or not to join the corps. Ph.D.s could opt instead to become research fellows, a position that was free of any hint of militarism but carried lesser benefits and lower pay.

Joel Montgomery, the microbiologist who had wrestled with Komodo dragons for his doctoral research, had donned the uniform without experiencing much culture shock. "Being a member of the Public Health Service is already significant, so why not wear the uniform," he said.

The thirty-two-year-old scientist, who for efficiency wore his blond hair in a short military-style cut, had taken to the uniform without difficulty in part because he was used to seeing it. He had spent the two years before EIS as a postdoctoral fellow in the parasitic diseases lab, which was tucked into the CDC's Chamblee site in northeast Atlanta. The stint had given him some familiarity with CDC culture, even though Chamblee was one of the offices where staff were least likely to wear the uniforms voluntarily. The sprawling fifty-acre campus, which had started life as a World War II Army hospital, was home to the National Center for Environmental Health. The center was infamous within the agency for its aging buildings, including some of the long-dismantled hospital's sixty-year-old wooden barracks. Termites regularly swarmed in several of the offices. In one lab, a scientist had rigged a $20 combination of duct tape, gutters, and a five-gallon bucket to keep air-conditioning condensation from dripping onto a $300,000 gas chromatograph.

Many of the environmental scientists were quirky specialists, nationally recognized experts in narrowly defined fields. More than a few of them came to work at night because the daytime fluctuations of the aging air-conditioning system disrupted the analyses they were running. Military customs and courtesies were not high on their to-do lists.

Montgomery, who already had more than ten years' experience as a bench scientist, had picked up some of the Chamblee attitude. Unless dignitaries were visiting, corps members could choose one of several uniforms to wear. He had opted for the least flamboyant: a set of almost-black trousers, long-sleeved shirt, and narrow tie that EIS members called the Johnny Cash Memorial Uniform. (The short-sleeved, all-khaki summer version was the UPS Driver; the uncomfortable, polyester-heavy dress whites were known as the Good Humor Man.)

He had experienced his own version of culture shock, though—not at the CDC, but once he ventured outside the lab.

For his EIS assignment, he had chosen work in the Special Pathogens Branch, part of the National Center for Infectious Diseases, the CDC's biggest division. As a title, "special pathogens" was a marvel of bureaucratic blandness masking the most potentially hazardous work done at the CDC. Special Pathogens' purview was highly infectious viruses that caused meningitis, encephalitis, and viral hemorrhagic fevers, including Ebola, newly discovered Nipah virus, and Rift Valley fever.

Special Pathogens were a small group, more male than female, who were accorded unusual respect within the CDC. Their public image was rule-flouting cowboys, an epidemiologic version of fighter pilots. In reality, they were more like test pilots: highly competent, undramatic people who understood that uncertainty was part of the job but had no interest in taking more risks than necessary. Their particular domain was a cream and blue building not far from the main gate that had extra layers of security—electronic locks, sign-in sheets, and guards—at all its doors. Inside, there were offices and normal bench space, and also the lab-within-a-lab—the "hot zone"—where the most infectious viruses were handled. The lab operated at the highest level of biosafety, four on a scale that went from one to four—a level reserved for exotic organisms that caused life-threatening disease, could be spread through the air, and could not be prevented by a vaccine. Working inside the zone required spacesuit-like protective gear, a contained air supply, and an end-of-shift dousing in a disinfectant shower.

One of the organisms that Special Pathogens studied was hantavirus, a pathogen carried by the kind of rodents—voles, mice, Norway rats—that like to live close to humans. Hantaviruses had been known for decades in Asia for causing hemorrhagic fevers, which are severe combinations of high fever, low blood pressure, bleeding through the walls of blood vessels, and shock. The first hantavirus isolated, in Korea in 1978, had turned out to be the cause of the 1951 epidemic that alarmed Alexander Langmuir and spurred the EIS's founding. In 1993, hantavirus had shown up in United States in a new guise: It caused a fast-moving pneumonia that sickened forty-eight people in the rural Southwest, killing twelve of them. Since then, investigators had kept a wary eye on the pathogen's movement through the Americas. By the beginning of 2002, there had been more than 1,200 cases of the newly recognized hantavirus pulmonary syndrome in the United States, Canada, and eight South American countries.

In late summer 2002, the Bolivian Ministry of Health notified the CDC that it had uncovered two cases of hantavirus pulmonary syndrome only a few hundred kilometers apart. One man, a physician who lived on a ranch, had survived; the other, a sugarcane cutter, had died. In the five years before that, there had been only eleven cases in the entire country. Special Pathogens sent eight people, including Joel Montgomery, to investigate.

By the time they arrived, the surviving case had recovered, and there was no sign of an outbreak. That was fine, since shutting down an epidemic was not the point of the trip. The investigators were looking instead for how widely the disease had spread in Bolivia. That required finding not only humans who might have been infected, but the disease hosts who had infected them. In other words, mice. The team needed to trap—and bleed, autopsy, and freeze—dozens of them.

"Ultimately you want to prevent this disease, but you can't do that until you know its basic biology in an area," Joel said. "We just don't know what the real prevalence of disease in those areas is."

"Those areas" were wide stretches of sugarcane fields in northeastern Bolivia. It took days to get there: Ten hours on paved road and twelve more on dirt roads, bumping along in cushion-free military Humvees loaned by a U.S. Navy research station. Their destination was three settlements where farm workers lived: a slum on the outskirts of an agricultural town, a settlement that subsistence farmers had carved out of the sugar fields, and rows of shacks built by migrant workers following the cane harvest.

It was Joel's first time in the field for the CDC. That part was thrilling: improvising a field lab, designing a solid study, going door-to-door in a barrio to persuade people to donate blood samples. The conditions, though, were deeply troubling—"deplorable" was the word Joel used.

The field workers' average wage was six dollars a day for cutting two tons of sugarcane. They worked every day of the week. They lived in clusters of shelters made of wood posts and blue tarps. The shacks were crammed full of cots and bunks, cobbled together out of sticks and rope. Some of the men had wives and children with them. Others were by themselves. They would crowd into the shacks, ten or more at a time, to sleep or take shelter from rainstorms and the winds whipped up by fires that cleared the fields of the cane stubble the cutters left behind. The shacks were pitched next to whatever water sources they could find in the fields—a water hole, or a slow-moving river where they washed, drank, and scooped water for cooking. Their health was terrible. They lived, on average, no more than forty-four years.

"We knew we were going to the poorest country in South America," Joel said. "But it was worse than I thought it would be. The way the migrants live is a human-rights nightmare."

Joel had started his EIS year wanting to get out from behind the microscope, into the human world of disease. The first foray had left him unexpectedly shaken.

———

Joel had been married for ten years to Kim, a special-education teacher. They met when he was an undergraduate at Texas A&M University. She had started out designing and programming phone systems for corporations, a lucrative job that helped defray the cost of Joel's graduate degrees. When he was done, she had switched to special ed; she was an in-school coach and companion to a girl with Down syndrome who was being mainstreamed in a suburban school system. It was much less stressful than her old job, and the hours were more reasonable. They were thinking it might be time to start a family.

Among veterans, the CDC had a reputation as a family-friendly employer. Most of the employees were married; remarkably for a place full of ambitious medical researchers, most of them were still married to the spouses they had met in graduate school twenty years before. Senior staff who had dragged wives or husbands to remote postings, or borne their children while on assignment in the developing world, made a point of being flexible when younger workers needed time off to pump breast milk or fetch a sick toddler from kindergarten. There was a moderately affordable day care across the street from the main gate. After the thirty-six-hour shifts of residency and the front-line rigors of the Peace Corps or Doctors Without Borders, the EIS felt like a relatively safe, stable place to raise a child.

Or so it seemed, going in. But by November, the officers with young children were finding that juggling home schedules, long work hours, and last-minute deployments was more challenging than they had imagined. They were, they thought, prepared to handle national emergencies. What they had not anticipated was the day-to-day work-load of their jobs.

"I knew that joining the Public Health Service and the EIS would mean being on call 24/7," said Karen Broder, a pediatrician with two toddlers who was married to a professor competing for tenure at Emory University, next door to the CDC. "What I didn't expect is that your significant other is on call 24/7 also. We factor it into every deci-sion we make now, whether it's his accepting an invitation to give a paper or our planning a family vacation."

Jennifer Gordon Wright, a veterinarian married to a landscape ar-chitect and who had been in private practice and public health gradu-ate school before she joined the corps, had her first child two months before EIS began. Jennifer was a calm, friendly woman with shoulder-length dark-blonde hair; she seldom seemed rattled by work, but combining corps service and child rearing taxed her usually posi-tive outlook. She had put the baby, Lauren, into her first day of day care on the first day of training; on the way, Lauren had thrown up on Jennifer's new and only uniform. Since then, she had been sent out of town twice: to western Virginia to monitor the human health risks of a raccoon-rabies vaccination program, and to the Caribbean to board a cruise ship blitzed by an outbreak of gastrointestinal viruses. Each time, she came back with suitcases of data to be analyzed.

"Day care closes at 6:30 p.m., and there were times during the out-break in September when I would be scrambling to get out of the of-fice, thinking I would find her on the doorstep," she said.

The officers had vowed, usually to themselves but occasionally out loud, that they would pay at least as much attention to their kids' needs as they would to their own professional satisfaction. It was a desirable goal but a practical day-to-day struggle. Seeing the others navigate the same difficulties made it only a little easier. Katrina Kretsinger, a physician assigned to foodborne illnesses who had three children under the age of four, sneaked back to her office one night after her kids had gone to sleep, to finish a report. Coming out of her office at 1:30 in the morning, she ran into Karen, who had done the same thing.

"There was one moment—and it hasn't been the only one—when I realized how hard this is to balance," Karen said. "I was pulling an all-nighter, to get a presentation ready that I hadn't had much time to work on. It was due at eleven a.m. the next day. And then my husband reminded me that it was our turn for kindergarten snack in the morning. So I went out to the store, got the snack, set it all up, and then came back and finished my project. That was when I realized that the minute daily things, which should be so easy to work into your life, turn out to be more challenging than the actual work you are doing."

The women had all sailed through medical training, a crucible for learning to manage multiple tasks on little sleep. They had expected EIS, with its extreme time demands, to feel like residency, and were taken aback to find it was worse. With several months' experience, they had begun to develop coping strategies. When day care deadline approached each day, Jennifer forwarded her work files to her home computer so she could pick up after dinner. Katrina began keeping memory books for all three children; the albums were a place to record small events that they would not remember and her overtired brain could not hold. Karen, who was small and slender and passionate about exercise, had started getting on her home stationary bike at 11:30 at night. She struck deals with her supervisor, shifting some workdays later in the day so she could work in one son's school store for an hour and accompany a class on a field trip to a petting zoo. (The previous year, the CDC had warned that petting zoos exposed children to hazardous bacteria. She made certain the entire class washed their hands.)

The one variable they could not plan for was the possibility of real hazard. Their bioterror training, coupled with the smallpox vaccination campaign, had unnerved them all.

"I don't feel entitled to put myself in danger," Jennifer said. "Before Lauren was born, I might have been more willing to go on a risky assignment. But now I don't want to put myself at risk, because she deserves to grow up with two parents."

Karen had taken an assignment in vaccine-preventable diseases because as a pediatrician she worried about the public backlash against vaccines. She had volunteered to work on the smallpox campaign, developing elaborate flowcharts intended to help doctors accurately diagnose a case of smallpox if they ever saw one. The poster-sized charts were highly detailed, studded with full-color pictures of florid smallpox and boxes of densely packed data. For more than a month, she hauled drafts back and forth between her office and her house, to work on late at night.

One evening, she was reading her five-year-old a story about a girl who tries to escape school by inventing illnesses: measles and mumps and stomachache and chickenpox, which all go away when the weekend arrives. He interrupted her.

"Mommy," he said, "you work on pox, don't you?"

Karen said she did.

"And it isn't chickenpox, is it?" he said.

Karen said no, it wasn't chickenpox; it was smallpox, a different disease.

"Can I get smallpox?" he asked.

She told him no.

"We had a talk," she said later. "He knows about vaccinations, so I explained that he didn't need the smallpox vaccine. That smallpox was something that happened a long time ago, and Mommy was just working on it to make sure it didn't happen again.

"You think about all the things you are going to need to talk about with your children," she said. "I never imagined that I would have to talk to a clinician about the difference between chickenpox and smallpox, let alone that I would have to talk about it to my own five-year-old child."

———

If the possible dangers of EIS service seemed unpredictably close for most of the class, they were especially acute for Scott Filler and Sami Gottlieb. They were the only ones who could not feel secure that, whatever risks they took, their spouse would be relatively safe. It made them look twice at what had seemed the perfect arrangement: the chance, for the first time in their eight years together, to work in the same institution at the same professional stage.

It was close to Christmas. They had both been home since early November and Scott was not scheduled to leave again until January. Sami was not yet visibly pregnant, but they had told a few colleagues. Their classmates were not only thrilled, but smug: In a contest held the last night of summer training, the couple had been voted "Most Likely to Have a Baby While in EIS."

The pregnancy made them both ineligible to volunteer for smallpox vaccination: Sami because the live virus in the vaccine might affect the baby, and Scott because he might accidentally pass the virus on to her. It was also affecting their planning, and not just for timing the CDC's maximum six weeks of maternity leave. Having a new baby would mean that only one of them at a time could leave town for an outbreak; Scott was already gone so frequently that Sami could foresee problems fitting her epidemic investigations in between his trips.

More subtly, the recognition that they were about to be a family had sharpened the care with which they examined each other's potential assignments for unrecognized risks. Sami was unsure whether to be more concerned about a deliberately caused hazard such as smallpox, or a naturally occurring new one such as Ebola. There was no vaccine for Ebola, and EIS members had been sent to investigate it several times. Scott—who had kept a before-marriage promise to give up extreme sports including ice climbing and paragliding—worried about more prosaic dangers: riots, gunfire, kidnapping. Earlier in the fall, one of their classmates had been in Ivory Coast when a coup started. She had returned unharmed, but it nagged at him that countries where he might be called to work could be politically unstable. With preparations mounting for war with Iraq, his disquiet increased.

"I have been scared about being overseas if war breaks out," he said. "There are a lot of us in remote areas. Should we stay where we are, try to get home, head for an embassy? No one has said."

The underlying fear, unspoken but potent, was that they would lose track of each other in an emergency. It would be surprisingly easy to do. Their jobs were on separate campuses that lay more than ten miles apart on roads covered by dense traffic. The only time they were likely to be in the same building was during a mandatory meeting every Tuesday morning, when EIS members who had completed investigations presented their findings to their classmates as a training exercise. And if a crisis came, things would move very quickly: On September 11, 2001, the first two EIS members dispatched to New York left within hours of the attacks, when most of the agency, and the country, were still reeling. And Scott and Sami both recognized the pressure to work that they were likely to impose on themselves.

"The one weekend that I came back during listeria—that fateful weekend—I was completely torn," Sami said. "Because I wanted so much to see him, but I needed every moment that I had. He was at a barbecue with our classmates, and I'd get these cell phone calls from him, and I'd be, just, begging: 'I just need one more hour . . .' "

Their greatest worry, they both said, was that if a crisis came, they might not be able to face the risks together.

"If something happened, they would have to put us together—not necessarily to work side by side, but to be in the same place," Scott said. "I wouldn't want to feel like you were somewhere completely different, where I couldn't reach you."

"If something happened, of course we would want to work on it," Sami agreed. "That's part of why we are here; that's part of what makes the job so interesting and exciting. But we would have to be together. That is not negotiable."

EIGHT

War

1994, Zaire

IN THE BELLY OF A C-130 CARGO PLANE, Don Sharp hunched over his duffel bags and waited for a signal.

It was very loud in the cavernous back of the airplane, and very dark. They had been flying for more than an hour. They were descending into a small airport north of Goma, Zaire, a few miles from the western border of Rwanda. Once, Goma had been a second-rate resort, a small town with a spiderweb of streets that was popular with Belgian tourists nostalgic for the wildness of their former colonial possession. Now it was a death zone. In the past ten days, almost 1 million refugees had poured through its streets and into the countryside, fleeing the Rwandan genocide. Cholera had struck, and measles and dysentery. Thousands of refugees were dying every day.

The pilot had explained the situation before they took off from Entebbe airport in Uganda. Goma's airport was in chaos, he said. There was no air traffic control and no one in charge. Cargo planes from a half-dozen nations were landing every hour with relief supplies, so heavily laden that the runway's tarmac was cracking and breaking up under the load. But there was not enough cargo-handling equipment to move the bundles rapidly, and there were robbers and rogue militiamen lurking on the borders of the airport, eager to seize whatever could be pried loose and carried away.

If the plane stopped to let them off, the pilot had said, the thieves might swarm the aircraft. So it was not going to stop. When they touched down in Goma, he told Sharp and the others, he would slow down as rapidly as possible, veer off the runway into a dirt area alongside, and hit the release button that opened the huge loading doors under the tail. Then, he said, they would jump from the moving airplane to the ground. As soon as he could see they were clear of the belly, he would shove the throttles forward and take off as fast as possible.

They might want to crouch down when they hit, the pilot added helpfully; it would protect them from flying gravel, and keep their bags from blowing away in the engines' exhaust. Once the plane was airborne, though, it would be a good idea to get into shelter quickly. Another plane would be coming close behind them.

Sharp, a former Navy submariner, had listened to the plan with disbelief. That had been several hours ago, in late afternoon. Goma was so dangerous that the pilots had not wanted to land after dark, but takeoff in Uganda had been delayed twice for mechanical problems, and it was dark now. The sky around the airport was lit with moving stars, the belly lights of more aircraft waiting for their chance to land and be off again.

The plane's wheels touched the fractured tarmac. It lurched as the speed brakes on the wing engaged, and the group in the back braced themselves, clinging to cargo webbing and the metal edges of the canvas benches along the sides of the fuselage. The nose swerved sharply as the pilot guided the craft to one side. The hydraulic hinges on the cargo hatch squealed behind them; the huge door separated slowly, extending a narrow metal ramp a few feet above the rapidly receding ground.

"Hit it!" the pilot yelled over his shoulder.

Sharp and his colleagues grabbed their bags, skidded to the edge, and jumped. They hit the packed earth, curling over the duffels and shielding their faces. Behind them, the plane swerved back to the runway, and the engines roared to life again.

They stood up, hitching the straps of their bags over their shoulders and peering through the dark for a way across the airfield. The dirt alongside the runway was heaped with crates and boxes that were stacked on top of each other and strapped onto pallets and huge rolling carts. The piles made a maze of twisting paths that led to the airport's small terminal buildings. Somewhere beyond them was the road into Goma.

The background noise of engines got suddenly louder. Sharp looked behind them. It was a 707, a cargo jetliner much bigger than the plane they had just jumped out of, and it was taxiing straight for them. He could see the co-pilot leaning out of the right-hand window, squinting to look beyond the pools of light cast by the taxi lights on the undercarriage. The nose of the plane twisted back and forth as the pilot sought the runway.

The CDC team were well beyond the edge of the light. The pilots would never see them in time. Next to them, a pallet of cargo began to rock, caught by the edge of the turning exhaust.

They ran.

―――――

Three months earlier, Rwanda had imploded.

The necessary conditions for the conflagration had been simmering for years. The tiny territory, whose name for itself was Ruanda-Urundi, had been colonized by the Germans and then taken away from them in the redivision of power that followed the end of World War I. Belgium inherited it and divided it into two, making the modern nations of Rwanda and Burundi. For centuries, Rwanda had been home to two major ethnic groups, the subsistence-farming Hutus and the cattle-herding Tutsis.

To solidify their control over the colony—a relative afterthought compared to the much larger and more fractious Belgian Congo next door, which would become Zaire—the Belgian colonial authorities formalized the ethnic division into a racial ideology. The Tutsi, who were thought to be taller and to have sharper facial features, were more "European," the colonialists decided, and therefore more deserving of social power than the stocky, broad-nosed Hutu. To reinforce the distinction, Belgian administrators created a system of national identity cards specifying which group the holder belonged to. The system ignored a fluid local understanding of identity—Hutu were allowed to "become" Tutsi if they gained sufficient cattle wealth—as well as generations of intermarriage between the groups, and it locked the Hutu majority into a position resembling that of serfs. Deepening the division between the groups, the colonial authorities proceeded to favor the Tutsis, whose hold on the monarchy and semifeudal aristocracy had survived the colonial transfer. For most of Belgian rule, only Tutsi were allowed to obtain higher education or hold lucrative government jobs.

The increasingly unstable system lasted for almost forty years. In 1957, the first opposition political group was formed: Parmehutu, the "party for the emancipation of the Hutu." The Belgian authorities— anticipating independence, and looking for a partner who would allow them to continue to profit from their about-to-be former colony—supported the restless majority. Then in 1959 the Tutsi king Rudigwa, who had reigned since being installed by the Belgians in 1931, died suddenly, and the Hutu rose in revolt. Thousands of Tutsi were massacred—estimates range from 10,000 to 100,000—and thousands more fled into Burundi, Uganda, and Zaire.

Rwanda's independence, under a Hutu president, was ratified by Belgium in 1962. Persecution of the Tutsi began; there were periodic massacres and purges. In 1973, a rival Hutu leader, Juvenal Habyarimana, took power in a coup. He set up a classically corrupt dictatorship, with a novel twist: The country's increasing poverty—caused by plundering by the political elite—was blamed on the now-oppressed Tutsi, who accounted for no more than 15 percent of the population.

In 1990, the Tutsi exiles struck back. A group called the Rwandan Patriotic Front (RPF)—who called themselves the "children of 1959" and were in many cases the literal children of those who had fled the uprising—crossed the border from Uganda. They fought their way well into the country, gaining support from moderate Hutu opposition to the Habyarimana government. After six months, unable to defeat the rebels, Habyarimana agreed to a cease-fire and to plans for multiparty power sharing. Simultaneously, though, his government began to train and indoctrinate an armed youth wing that carried the name Interahamwe, "those who attack together."

Power sharing was so slow in coming that international donors and the United Nations eventually forced the Rwandan government to the bargaining table. In August 1993, Habyarimana and the RPF signed an agreement for a multiparty government and repatriation of the exiles. The accord was furiously opposed by the Hutu elite, who viewed Habyarimana as a traitor. A new radio station, Radio Mille Collines, began broadcasting from the capital, Kigali, denouncing the agreement and vilifying the Tutsi. The station's owners were later revealed to be highly placed staff from the ministry of information and foreign ministry.

On April 6, 1994, the plane carrying Habyarimana back from an accord-related meeting was shot down as it returned to Kigali airport. The killing began immediately. Within hours, roadblocks were thrown up. The military went from house to house, slaughtering Hutu moderates and the few Tutsi in the capital. They knew where to find their victims, because the identity-card system—created by the Belgians and maintained by the Hutu government—provided an ethnic map to every neighborhood and household. And when people tried to escape, Radio Mille Collines foiled them: It broadcast the license plate numbers of cars owned by those the government wanted killed.

The military and Interahamwe brought the massacres to the countryside. Hate radio poured out propaganda, urging civilians to join the slaughter. They obeyed. Over the course of 100 days, more than 800,000 Tutsi and moderate Hutus were shot, bludgeoned, and hacked to death. They died in their homes, in schools, in churches where they had fled for sanctuary, and in fields where they were tracked down, running for their lives. They were killed not only by the militias, but by their doctors, pastors, neighbors, and friends.

Within days of Habyarimana's assassination, the RPF abandoned the cease-fire and counterattacked. On July 21, they declared victory. It was a hollow achievement: Seventy-five percent of the Tutsi population of Rwanda had been murdered, and the murderers were beyond the RPF's reach. Driving the Hutu population before them, and egging them on with hate-radio broadcasts predicting retaliatory slaughter by the Tutsis, the Rwandan government and at least 2 million of its Hutu citizens had fled the country.

The refugees in the camps in Goma, the ones the CDC had dispatched its team to help, were Hutu.

———

The refugees had begun pouring over the border into Goma on July 14. They overwhelmed the town, which lies just over the border on the north shore of Lake Kivu. Within days, Zairean authorities herded them out of the city, into flat fields that became makeshift squatter camps: Mugunga, eleven miles to the west, and Kibumba and Katale, fifteen and thirty-five miles to the north.

The refugees had left home with nothing, and the area around Goma had little to offer them. The town was at a high elevation, and cold at night. It lay on a volcanic plain with two active volcanoes to the north, covered by a thin crust of earth that sustained spindly trees. Where the lava was thick, there was no access to water. There was nothing to absorb the impact of 800,000 frightened, sick, and starving people.

On July 20, the first case of cholera was diagnosed in the camps. It spread with lightning speed. One week later, seven thousand people died of it in a single day.

The CDC had sent several teams to the emergency. One group had been inside Rwanda since June, including an EIS officer who worked in neighboring Burundi. Two other physicians had just left Atlanta. Bradley Woodruff, known as Woody, was with the CDC's refugee health branch; he had worked for a year in Kenya. Scott Dowell, a pediatrician, had been in the EIS for a year. When he was growing up, his father, also a pediatrician, had done volunteer medical work in Haiti and taken his family along. Dowell spoke fluent French, Rwanda's first language.

Then there was the group Sharp belonged to. He was forty-one, a physician who had been an undersea medical officer for four years and then gone to work for Kaiser Permanente in San Diego. That had paled quickly. He and his wife, a nurse practitioner he had met at Kaiser, had signed up with an international relief organization. They were posted to Pakistan's border with Afghanistan, to treat refugees and train Afghan combat medics. Then they went to Thailand for three years, caring for refugees in a resettlement camp 100 miles from Bangkok. Thailand was a rough assignment. Sharp's first patient there had a live cockroach wedged firmly against her eardrum, and the doctors on his team did more than 100 physicals a day, seeing malaria, dengue, typhus, and dysentery. Plus it was hazardous for a couple starting a family: Sharp's wife contracted dengue, was menaced by a cobra, and while she was pregnant with their first child was bitten by a dog and had to take rabies shots. But while they were there, Sharp met the CDC's representative in Asia, an international health veteran named Bob Keegan. Keegan told him about the EIS. Sharp applied from Thailand and, after being placed on the waiting list, was accepted and assigned to Missouri.

In the summer of 1994, Sharp had just graduated from EIS. He had opted for a third year of training at CDC headquarters, an option called the preventive medicine residency. On his first day of work, he found a note on his computer, asking him to return a phone call. He did. The voice on the other end said: "Can you get on a plane in two days and go to Zaire?"

There were six others in the team: three EIS officers—Orin Levine and Alfredo Vergara, both Ph.D.s, and Judith Moore, a nurse and midwife—and three CDC staff members: Peter Bloland, a veterinarian, and physicians Brent Burkholder and David Swerdlow, who had all been in the EIS three to five years earlier. Burkholder, who was the same age as Sharp and had also joined the CDC in mid-career, was in charge.

Sharp's group reached Entebbe, the closest international airport, on the morning of July 29. It was pouring rain when they landed. The airport was crowded and busy. International governments had ignored the Rwandan crisis while the genocide was going on—even the

United Nations had withdrawn most of the peacekeeping troops it had sent to monitor the start of power sharing—but with the emergency spilling past the borders, they had sprung into action. Given the crisis, there was no commercial air service to Goma. There were military flights, and private cargo haulers working for the UN and other agencies—and there were hundreds of relief workers, journalists, and military officers all vying to wedge themselves in amongst the relief supplies for the two-hour flight.

The team had known when they left Atlanta that they would have to improvise once they got to Entebbe. After a few hours there, they realized how challenging a task that would be. There was no space left in any of the planes going that day, and no promise of any the next day. Discouraged, they begged a box of Meals-Ready-to-Eat from a U.S. Army detachment, found a place to rest, and settled down to wait. The next day, they found a few seats on a military transport, enough to send the EIS officers and Peter Bloland on ahead.

It took another twenty-four hours for Sharp, Swerdlow, and Burkholder to find seats, and then four hours more while they shuttled between planes with mechanical problems. By the time they ran off the Goma tarmac, it was after 10:00 p.m. There was no sign of the other team members, and no vehicle looking for them from the office of the UN's High Commissioner for Refugees (UNHCR). But there were the robbers they had been warned about. In the glare of generator-driven work lights that had been hauled in by military detachments, the CDC people could see shadowy figures on the other side of the runway. They were running out from a stand of trees, hacking at the cargo webbing with long knives, and hauling off the boxes they had cut free.

The three doctors dragged their gear into a shadow behind one of the work lights and debated what to do. A different engine noise cut through the hubbub: A U.S. Army Humvee was skirting the cargo dump. They ran out from the shadows, waving. An Army logistics unit was camped at the north end of the airport, against a fence topped with razor wire; the driver agreed to take Burkholder to negotiate with their commander. Close to midnight, they returned. No one would be going into Goma that night—the unlit road was far too dangerous—but the team could bunk in a corner of a tent if they liked.

The next morning was more of the same: more planes, more reports of dangerous surroundings; no available rides into town, and no word from their CDC colleagues or UN hosts. Sharp was standing on the side of the runway, wondering what they should do next, when a pickup truck swerved by. On the side was the seal of the International Organization for Migration, one of the groups he had worked for in Thailand. In the passenger seat was Dr. Vince Keene, his former boss.

"I hadn't seen him in three years," Sharp said. "He was very casual. He said, 'Hey, doc, do you need a ride?' And I said, 'Well, Vince, that would be nice.' "

The truck took him into Goma, to where UNHCR had set up shop in a building abandoned by owners fleeing the cross-border chaos. At the offices, Sharp found the other half of the team, and a reception that none of them were expecting.

"What are you doing here?" one of the UNHCR representatives asked. "We have too many people already. We're not sure what to do with the ones who are here now."

Sharp found a taxi that would take him back to the airport to fetch Swerdlow and Burkholder. When the team reassembled, at a primitive hotel charging eye-gouging prices, they debated what to do next. They decided to stay.

———

The team began to explore Goma, to find ways they could be useful.

The first thing that met them was the smell. The second was the cause of the smell: the bodies. There were dead bodies on the verge of every road, lying alone, or piled into neat heaps. Most of the dead had been neatly wrapped in sarongs or sleeping mats by whoever had carried them to the roadside. Crews in borrowed trucks—soldiers, relief workers, and the Zairean Boy Scouts—roamed the roads, picking up the bodies and ferrying them west of town. There, the French Army had dug mass graves with backhoes. To save time, knowing that more graves would be needed, they blew the underlying lava apart with dynamite. The dynamiting threw a sharp black dust into the air that mixed with the smoke from cooking fires and the stench of the corpses.

On their first day in Goma, Sharp passed one end of the first mass grave.

"You could see clearly through the dirt: There was a foot; there was a head, an elbow," he said. "They were doing the best they could, but it was too hard to dig down deep."

In a cable to UNHCR headquarters, a UN representative described it: "Overwhelmed with deaths and suffering. . . . Site chaotic, unmanaged, unplanned. . . . Corpses everywhere."

The impenetrable lava that lay so close to the surface had contributed to the cholera epidemic. Cholera is a disease of poor sanitation; it strikes when people ingest food or water that is contaminated with sewage. The bacteria produce a toxin that disrupts the lining of the small intestine, pulling water from the tissues. The key feature of cholera is copious diarrhea that quickly becomes clear as the intestines empty. The body's fluid reserves pour out at a rate of a quart an hour or more, carrying essential minerals with them. Cholera dehydration can kill in less than a day. Once an outbreak begins in a population, cholera spreads explosively.

The prerequisites for controlling cholera are safely disposing of feces, and obtaining clean water for drinking and washing food. But the lava made those impossible: It was too thick to dig latrines or drill wells. Clean water is essential for taking care of victims as well. Cholera symptoms last three to five days; if victims take in as much fluid and salt as they are losing, they can survive until the attack exhausts itself. But clean water was unavailable in the camps. Because there were no wells, the refugees walked to Lake Kivu and carried water back to their families. But the lake water was not clean. The lake, which crossed the border into Rwanda, was loaded with decomposing bodies.

The CDC team could do little to halt the spread of the cholera outbreak, or the outbreak of shigella dysentery that followed it. They began looking for smaller tasks that they could manage.

There were an estimated 300,000 people in each camp, and UNHCR thought there might be 150,000 more squatting around Goma town. The camps were flat fields whose shallow crust of earth had been churned up by thousands of feet passing back and forth over it. In places, the sharp edges of old lava flows were exposed. In others, there were shoals of mud created by spilled water and sick people. With so few latrines—in Mugunga, there was one for every 1,200 people—the camps had become an open sewer.

The fields were not large, so the camps were crowded. The refugees were packed so tightly that when workers walked through the crowds, they had to be careful not to step on people's legs.

Some of the relief agencies had begun pitching tents in the camps, for clinics and food distribution centers. Some supplies had begun to arrive: antibiotics, tarpaulins, basic foods like flour and sugar. But the agencies had no way to gauge whether the supplies were being distributed efficiently. Alfredo Vergara adopted that as his job.

Vergara was a Chilean who had grown up in Venezuela. He had a Ph.D. in environmental and occupational health, but he wanted to do international work. He had been at the CDC for a year, assigned to the program that worked to prevent lead poisoning, and he had just returned from an assignment in the Angolan civil war.

He decided to focus on the refugees' nutrition. Most of them had little food and few possessions. After two weeks on the run, they looked like people who were hungry: They were listless and quiet, especially the children. People stood or squatted or lay down in the same space, day after day. It was important, he thought, to know what these refugees' situation was now, when the crisis was new. It would help the relief agencies to determine afterward whether they had made a difference. And it would indicate whether food was reaching the people who needed it, or was being diverted by bad management, or stolen and sold.

He used what was called a cluster-sample survey. He drew a map of each camp, divided them into rough geographic zones, and estimated the number of people in the zones by climbing high up in the surrounding hills so that he could look down on the crowds. For each camp, he chose thirty zones at random to focus on, and twenty family groups in each zone. The results gave him a cross-section of the camps' population that was random enough and numerous enough to be statistically valid.

He and his helpers picked their way through the areas they had selected, to find families to interview. They asked the adults how many of their group had died since they came to Zaire, whether they had been sick, whether they had shelter, and whether they had food or could get it from the relief agencies. They weighed the children who were younger than five years old, and measured their height.

They found what they expected to find: The refugees were going hungry. Almost one in four children was acutely malnourished, based on a comparison of their weight against their height, which was a good gauge of their age. But they also found something they did not expect. The malnutrition was not just because of the chaotic flight across the border. It was also due to a fault in the way the agencies were distributing food.

The camps had grown up so rapidly that the UN had no opportunity to create a registry of the inhabitants, a master document that would list everyone in a camp and their ages, genders, and family structure. That was standard practice in refugee relief—but the Goma situation was so beyond the standard that none of the usual strategies could be applied. Instead, the UN had decided to rely on the political structure the refugees had occupied in Rwanda. It identified community leaders, men who were heads of districts, and made them responsible for dividing the food supplies and passing them on to representatives of townships and family villages.

It was an acceptable work-around, but it had a serious flaw: The Rwandan political structure was the domain of men. Women had no standing. But many of the men were missing.

"There were a lot of families where the men had been killed in the fighting, or had died," Vergara said. "And in those families, the women and children were not getting any food."

———

The bodies by the roadsides had not all died of cholera, and they were not all composed and cared for. Every morning, there were corpses that sprawled messily across the ground as though they had been flung there. They were bloody, with deep machete wounds. And there was something else: They were tall. The hatred that had torn Rwanda apart had come with the refugees across the border.

There were murders in the camps every day. Some of them were over theft, though there were few things to steal—a blanket, a tarp, very occasionally a spare biscuit or stash of food.

"Early one morning, we had assembled a bunch of volunteers; we were starting a training for the survey," Vergara recalled. "And in the distance we saw a crowd, maybe a hundred people, chasing one man. And then just a little while later, we heard screams, and thuds. And no one said anything. There was nothing you could say. You just got on with your work."

The CDC team understood that theft was common in Goma. The refugees had so little that every scrap was precious. And civilization had dissolved in the camps. There was only one imperative: to ensure your family's survival, if they had made it this far; to keep yourself going, if they had not. But the events the Americans witnessed made it hard to believe that punishment was the sole reason behind the killings, unless the punishment was for a transgression quite different from theft.

A few days after arriving, Sharp began helping staff from the American Refugee Committee carry dehydrated refugees from their huts to the treatment tents. The ARC had a truck. They were driving down one of the roads between the camps when they spotted a commotion off to one side, next to a market that had sprung up. They pulled over. The roadbed was higher than the surrounding land, and it gave them a clear view of the group. In the center was a Rwandan who looked stunned and injured; he had been beaten, or perhaps stoned. He had been running away; that was the commotion they had seen. Now the group had him cornered. In the front of the crowd, a man lifted a machete and advanced on the victim. He hacked at him, forcing him down onto the ground, and then beheaded him.

As they drove away, two things stuck in Sharp's memory. The first was visual: The man had been very tall. Until he fell to the ground, the man with the machete had had to rise on his toes to strike him.

The second was a sound, the dull, ringing thud of a machete landing on bone.

The violence extended to the relief workers as well. An ARC crew was robbed, and their driver was beaten. Trucks were stolen. Supplies were taken: One Hutu militiaman appropriated bags of food by threatening the workers in a food distribution tent with a hand grenade. There were threats outside the camps also. On their third day in Goma, Sharp and Levine asked one of the UN drivers to take them down to Lake Kivu; they had heard there were small bands of refugees camped on the shore of the lake. Their car was stopped by a squad of Zairean military.

"They opened the door, sat down next to us in the car, and one of them put the barrel of his AK-47 up against my neck," Sharp said. "They were yelling at us to keep driving, yelling at the driver that we weren't supposed to be on that road. I thought, Well, it was a good life. And then they stopped us, and put their hands out for money. We found twenty bucks for them very fast."

Many of the refugees were not violent. Most were numb, traumatized by the rapid succession of civil war, dislocation, hunger, and illness. The conditions bred a blank indifference to their own fate, and to that of others. Vergara saw it when he walked the camps for his survey.

"We came upon a family that were grouped together around a fire, and there was a woman with a baby, lying to one side," Vergara said. "The woman was unconscious; she had cholera, she was lying in a pool of excrement and water. The baby was less than a year old, sitting next to her, crying and crying."

Vergara asked the family if the woman was with them. No, they said, she was not part of their group. They had nothing to do with her. Vergara was shocked.

"She was not attached to anyone, and no one was caring for her or her baby," he said. "She was dying there, and they were not concerned."

Sharp saw the same thing. UNHCR had asked him to launch a giant vaccination campaign to protect the refugees against measles, a frequently fatal disease in Africa, and polio and meningitis, which would spread easily in the camps' chaos. The job required moving in and out of all three camps and negotiating with relief agencies for personnel, supplies, and space, but the campaign was focused on Mugunga camp. Mugunga was where much of the military and

Interahamwe had fled. Many of them still wore their uniforms; their Jeeps and tanks were parked among the few trees at the edge of the camp that had not been torn down for firewood. Within the surrounding misery, they had created a privileged enclave: They had plenty of food, looted from the refugee groups' stores, piles of marijuana, and a still. They were usually drunk, frequently high, and always menacing. Relief workers avoided that part of the camp when they could.

Sharp could not. He was searching for sites for the vaccination campaign, so the refugees would not have to walk far from their family groups. Wherever he and his companions went, they found people too weak to walk who needed to be moved to the clinic tents. If they were transferred and given an IV quickly enough, they might survive.

"Some parts of the camp, you couldn't get a vehicle into, so anyone who had to be moved had to be carried out," he said. "A few times, we asked the young men in the camp to help us. They laughed at us."

Shortly, many of the charities decided they would no longer deal with adults, unless they were dying. They focused their efforts on the incontrovertible victims of the emergency: the children.

———

In the rush to the border, thousands of children had become separated from their families. In the Goma camps, there were more than ten thousand. Most of them had no idea where their parents were, or whether they were living. Many of them were too young to be able to say.

There were shelters in the camps where the children were being taken care of, run by refugee groups or by Zairean health care workers. The staff who ran the centers refused to call their charges "orphans"; instead, they used "unaccompanied minors," signaling a hope that their families might still be living somewhere, and that they might be united some day.

The death rate in the centers was high. In one, called Ndosho, 180 children died in a month, out of 2,200 living there; in another, Muungano, 49 children died out of 351. Most of the children were desperately sick, from cholera and starvation. Most of the people caring for them had little knowledge of how to do so. There were supplies; the United Nations Children's Fund had rushed them IVs and oral rehydration salts, two essentials for replacing the fluids and electrolytes lost to cholera diarrhea. But there was not always an explanation of how to use the supplies, and little time to learn: Each caretaker at the centers was in charge of about twenty kids.

Improving the care of the unaccompanied minors became Scott Dowell's job. He and Woodruff were working for UNICEF; they had arrived a few days before Sharp and Vergara's team. Dowell was sleeping on the stone floor of a UNICEF representative's hotel room. It was his first international assignment.

"We were there to help, but we weren't sure at first what we should be doing," he said. "So we started going around, and we found these unaccompanied children's camps. A lot of times it was just a corner of a field where they would set up some tents, and the kids would come and then more and more kids would come. Within twelve hours of opening one of these things, there would be one hundred, two hundred kids. Sometimes infants with no parents. No food. No shelter. And bad diarrhea, a lot of them."

Caring for the children was not easy. Children need fluids to survive cholera, just as adults do. When it worked, hydration was magical: A child would go from listless and concave to bright-eyed and plump within hours. But the process of hydration was sensitive. Whether they were given by mouth or through an IV, the fluids needed a precise balance of salts and minerals. And they needed to be given slowly; too much would overwhelm a child's failing kidneys and kill as quickly as the cholera would.

It was a subtlety that had not been communicated to the workers caring for the children. They were well-intentioned and very dedicated, and many of them were malnourished and sick themselves. But they were overwhelmed. In the centers—many of which were merely tents—it was common to find eight or ten toddlers lying crosswise on an Army cot, with IV lines dangling overhead. The cots sagged in the middle, forcing the children in the center to lie in a pool of muck. Usually, when Dowell went into a center, two or three children would be dead. By the time he had made the rounds of the room, another would have died.

One day Dowell helped move cots in one of the centers, to make room for some adults who were coming to be taught about hydration. In one of the blankets, he found a body: a five-year-old child who had been dead about twenty-four hours.

Dowell and Woodruff calculated the mortality rate in the centers, using a standard epidemiological measure of a ratio with a denominator of 10,000. In the centers caring for toddlers, the rate went from 10 to 59. In the ones caring for infants, the rate started at 226 and went as high as 817.

"We would come up to these centers in the morning and see a little pile of what looked like firewood outside the entrances," he said. "It was the bodies of the kids who had died during the night. They would wrap the bodies up in blankets and tie them with string, and leave them by the door for the trucks to come and pick up."

Dowell had just finished his pediatric residency. Mixing a rehydration solution, calculating the right amount of fluid to give, and even cutting down to find a usable vein for an IV were familiar tasks to him. He set out to teach the same skills—or at least explain the priorities—for as many child caregivers as he could.

"We would go into a center and find kids lying on the floor, severely dehydrated, with a clogged IV," he said. "And then we would go outside and find the relief workers building a stone fireplace, so the kids could have hot meals in a few days. And we'd have to say, Hot meals would be great, but in a few days you're not going to have any living kids to cook meals for. You need to stop doing this. You need to take this oral rehydration solution and sit by this child and spoon it into his mouth, right now. Do it for the next three hours. Don't do anything else, or this child is going to be dead."

By the end of August, the death rates in the centers for unaccompanied children dropped to one-sixth of what they had been in July. It signaled both the passing of the cholera epidemic and the centers' belated success in nurturing and feeding children.

Most of the CDC staff left Goma as August ended. A few of them felt that, amidst the chaos, they had created something positive.

"There are few situations where you can feel you have an immediate impact," Dowell said. "This was one of mine."

It is likely that Dowell's coaching of the center staffs through the way to treat cholera victims saved some children's lives, possibly hundreds of lives. Vergara, whose sleuthing in the camps made it possible for women and children to be fed, felt the same way.

"It is not always the case, with the work you do, that you see a result immediately," he said. "A lot of the time you produce a long-term effect, or a diffuse one, or one that only improves things for a small population. But in this case, what we did saved lives right away."

But they remained haunted by the reality of who it was they had helped: those who had perpetrated the genocide, or abetted it, or acquiesced to it.

"When I walked around the camps, I would see a soldier staring at me, and know that a few weeks before, this person had had a machete in their hands," Sharp said. "But when you saw the conditions they were living in now—well, maybe someone could remain unmoved by it, but I couldn't. I couldn't condemn them. They were already in a hell on earth."

It was common, in EIS work, for officers to feel like visitors in the lives of others, bit players in a history that would continue long after they had stepped offstage. Succeeding at the job required becoming comfortable with never knowing how the story ends. The Goma team found that harder than most. Almost ten years later, they still thought about the camps, and wondered about the fate of the people they had treated there.

Scott Dowell now works for the CDC in Bangkok. On a wall in his house, there hangs a picture of one of the children in one of the centers for unaccompanied minors in Goma. The boy is no more than two years old. He looks healthy. His head has been shaved, and there is a strip of masking tape across his forehead. On the tape, a name is written: Simbizi. It is the name the center staff made up for him; he was too young to tell them what his real name was, and the only people who might have known were absent, or dead.

"He followed me around the center," Dowell said. "Some of the kids would tug on your pants, or touch you. He just stared at me, and he followed me around.

"I hope that a lot of those children were adopted, or found their way back to their families," he said. "But I don't know what happened to any of them. My wife often asks me what I think happened to Simbizi. But I have nothing to go on. I don't even really know his name."

NINE

Malaria

March 2003, Malawi

THE GUESTS WHO SAT CRAMMED against the walls of the four-room hut could hear the procession coming before they saw it. Sonorous hymns, long lines of praise in complex multipart harmonies, gusted through the unglazed windows along with the misty rain. The singers paced slowly into view: Eight women from the tiny Christian church in the closest village, wearing white blouses, navy-blue skirts and flip-flops that stuck in the churned-up mud of the dooryard. The first woman in the line carried a large cross in front of her, woven from dried grass and purple bougainvillea. Behind the last woman came the ministers, wearing brilliant red plastic ponchos over Roman collars and damp black robes.

The funeral was so well attended that only close relatives and important guests could be shoehorned into the mud-brick house. The rest stood outside, segregated into groups of men and women and clustered under umbrellas and tree branches that provided a little shelter from the rain. The two ministers took up positions on the deep open porch, setting their hard-soled shoes carefully on the slick surface of the earth berm that held up the house. One of them, a tall man with wire-rimmed glasses and bicycle clips still hanging from his trouser cuffs, opened a Bible. "Psalm 22," he announced in English. Switching to Chichewa, the main language of Malawi, he sang out the first line: "My God, my God, why hast thou forsaken me?"

From under the trees, the entire congregation answered him. "Why art thou so far from helping me?" they sang in intricate harmony. "I cry by day, but thou dost not answer; and by night, but find no rest."

In the small room at the front of the house, Scott Filler shifted discreetly. The family had put him in a place of honor: He was sitting on a dried-grass mat against an interior wall, facing the windows and with a clear view of the service outside. Still, the unfurnished room was so crowded that the only way to accommodate everyone was to sit straight up with legs straight out in front, a common posture in rural Malawi but hard to take for a Westerner whose hamstrings were unused to it. Anything more than a tiny movement, and someone would notice—either the tall woman nursing a baby tucked in on his left, or the nurse wedged in to his right, who was weeping and blotting her eyes with the cloth of her skirt. The funeral was for the father of Kingston Bulala, the chief lab technician in the project that had brought Filler to Malawi. Diplomacy and decorum required that he wait out the lengthy service without flinching or drawing attention to himself.

It was the end of the wet season in Malawi. Runoff from daily thunderstorms had cut deep channels into the unpaved roads that led up the hills to the Bulala family compound, three tin-roofed huts tucked into a cornfield behind a huge brick cistern. It was the family's second attempt at a funeral. The day before, the incessant rain had filled the freshly dug grave and collapsed it. Neighbors had come to keep the widow company, sitting by the body while they waited for the rain to stop. They clustered in the back room with her, sobbing in a rhythmic alto counterpoint to the minister's rumbling bass.

The senior Mr. Bulala, a man in his fifties, had been ill for a while. No one was willing to say what caused his death. That was not uncommon in Malawi, a southern African country that is one of the world's poorest. One out of every six Malawians was thought to be infected with HIV; in the past few years, so many adults had died that almost half of the population was children younger than fifteen. AIDS killed directly, and it made infected people vulnerable to other deadly illnesses: malaria, tuberculosis, schistosomiasis, and bacterial infections. Yet HIV and AIDS remained a taboo subject; even to raise the possibility was considered deeply impolite. Mr. Bulala might have died of heart disease, friends had said in the Jeep on the way to the funeral; he might have had diabetes. They had spoken with a shrug of discomfort, sliding their eyes away to watch goats pick their way through the rain.

The funeral was over. The choir had finished with Psalm 91: "You will not fear the terror of the night, nor the arrow that flies by day, nor the pestilence that stalks in darkness." The guests gathered slowly, picking up shoes and umbrellas from the porch and forming a line at one side of the dooryard. The sobs in the back room rose to a choking wail. Around the corner of the house, four men carried a simple coffin of sanded bare wood with hammered tin handles. The ministers and choir took their places in front of it, and the column moved off in silence. As they entered the narrow track through the cornfield, the sun broke through the trees.

Filler watched them go. "Well," he said, "another day in the life of an EIS officer."

———

AIDS had not brought Filler to Malawi. Malaria had. The thirty-three-year-old internist had been fascinated by the disease since college for a very personal reason: It had almost killed him.

"I had two undergraduate majors—applied mathematics and biology—and I spent a year in Kenya to do biology studies," he said. "At the tail end of the trip, I caught cerebral malaria. I was really sick; in two weeks I lost thirty-five pounds. I was on a small island off the coast, very remote, and a doctor from India happened to be traveling through the village I was in. Cerebral malaria is a really bad disease, but he knew what to do. He saved my life."

The rescue left Filler intrigued by medicine, but he did not follow the leaning immediately. After graduating from Brown, he went back to San Francisco where he had grown up. He left biology behind and went to work for a strategic management consulting firm.

"I did think about going to medical school," he said. "But I was just done with undergrad and I needed to pay off my loans. So I was a consultant for two years. In the end, I realized I liked the lifestyle but I didn't like the life. So I sent out applications to medical school, and while I was waiting to hear, I moved to Colorado and became a snowboarding instructor."

His highly nonstandard background caught the eye of the medical school admissions committee at University of California-San Francisco. In the spring of his first year at UCSF, a third-year resident walked into the section of the medical library where Filler was studying. She was on call and due back on the hospital's surgical service in four hours; she was looking for a quiet place to nap.

She never got the nap. The resident was Sami Gottlieb. The two started dating before the academic year ended. They were three years apart in age but six years apart in schooling, a huge gulf in medical training because it spans most of the journey from neophyte to physician.

"It was harder on Sami, I think," Filler said, "because she had already gone through the entire process of med school and residency. Probably the last thing she wanted was to go through it again."

Against the odds, the couple lasted, possibly because they spent so little professional time together. While Scott was in school, Sami was a professor; when he became a resident, she did research and studied for another degree. They agreed that, once Scott's training was done, the next move would be Sami's. If she made it into the EIS, they would relocate to Atlanta.

The couple had promised themselves a present: Once both were finished, they would take a year off together. In the summer of 2001, they left for South America and then Southeast Asia. To break up the trip, they stopped for six weeks in Hanoi to work for the CDC's global AIDS program, evaluating the clinical care of HIV patients in a country that has rapidly improving hospitals but not enough money to afford sophisticated drug regimens.

The trip gave Scott a chance to reflect. He had gotten a public health degree during training, a diploma awarded by the London School of Tropical Medicine and Hygiene after a four-month course, but he had little interest in U.S. public health. His interests lay overseas, and malaria still tugged at his attention. Getting a close look at a CDC international program suggested to him that there might be more than one way to go abroad.

"If Sami got into EIS, I thought we would go to Atlanta and I would work in clinical medicine for two years and build up our finances," Scott said. "But when she started doing her application and I read the materials, I thought it looked exciting. I figured, if I was moving to Atlanta anyway, I might as well try to get in too."

He succeeded, landing a job in the epidemiology division of the malaria branch, exactly where he had hoped to be. Ten days after starting work there, he left on his first international assignment to the Philippines, to give advice on the country's method of tracking malaria cases. His supervisor accompanied him to make introductions and get the project started, but four days later Scott was on his own.

"It was exactly what I wanted to be doing," he said. "We were going out to villages, me and a driver and a representative from the ministry of health, talking to people about how they were diagnosed for malaria and how they got drugs for it. One day, though—we were on Mindanao, in the southern Philippines—the ministry representative got a text message on his beeper. The ministry thought we should break off our trip. There had been some Abu Sayyaf guerrilla activity in the next village we planned to visit, five kilometers away."

They scrambled to change their plans, driving out of the remote village that night and leaving the island the next morning. When they returned to Manila, they discovered what guerrilla "activity" meant. The group had kidnapped two nurses working for an international health organization, and beheaded them.

The work in the Philippines was a foretaste of the main job the malaria branch had set aside for Scott. He was to run a clinical trial of malaria treatment in Malawi, a country so little known that, when he announced he was going, most of his friends had to look it up.

———

For someone fascinated by malaria, Africa is an ideal destination, if "ideal" can be applied to a disease that infects 300 million people and kills 1 million of them every year. Up to 90 percent of those deaths happen in sub-Saharan Africa, and most of them are children younger than five.

Malaria is uniquely dangerous to pregnant women and their infants. In areas where malaria-carrying mosquitoes bite year-round, people develop some immunity to the disease, though the protection takes years to build up and is never absolute. But women who are immune to malaria lose the protection when they become pregnant. Malaria in pregnancy can cause high fever and anemia, conditions that trigger miscarriage and premature delivery. As the parasite reproduces in a pregnant woman's system, it clusters in the blood vessels of the placenta, blocking the flow of oxygen and nutrients to the fetus and inhibiting its development. The result, if the fetus survives, is a child that weighs too little at birth. In the developing world, low birth weight is one of the most common reasons for children dying before their first birthday.

Studies done by the CDC more than ten years earlier showed that giving women two doses of an antimalarial drug during pregnancy could prevent the disease even in areas where malaria was common, potentially saving both mother and child. The vehicle for getting the drug to women was prenatal clinics. Even in very rural parts of Africa, more than two-thirds of women make the trip to a local clinic several times before they deliver. But there were limits to when the drug most used against malaria in Africa—sulfadoxine-pyrimethamine, usually called SP—could be given. Taken too early in the first trimester, it could cause spina bifida; taken too close to delivery, it caused a neonatal jaundice that could lead to brain damage.

It was hard, in the African rural clinics, to tell exactly when was too early or too late. Village nurses, lacking Western technology, estimated the age of the fetus by measuring the fundal height, the distance from the mother's pubic bone to the top of the uterus. In general, every extra centimeter equals another week of pregnancy. But fundal height is a rough gauge, and the estimates of age it yields can be off by several weeks. In addition, village women frequently could not say precisely when they became pregnant; their own guesses of how far along they were could differ from the nurses' estimates by three weeks or more. The discrepancies narrowed the window in which it was safe to give antimalarials. A woman who thought she was entering her third trimester could come to a clinic for her second dose and be told she was too far along for the drug to be safe.

In a CDC study done in Malawi in 2000, 95 percent of pregnant women visited a prenatal clinic at least twice, but only 35 percent succeeded in getting both doses of SP. At the same time, a second study demonstrated how rising rates of AIDS were complicating the situation: Pregnant women who were HIV-positive were not protected against malaria until they received a third dose of drugs.

Working with the World Health Organization and the Malawian Ministry of Health, the CDC decided to try a new tack. It would attempt to get women to take a dose every month of their pregnancies, aiming for at least three doses but hoping for four or five. Because the regimen would be more complicated and more expensive, and had never been tried on a significant scale, the agency planned a study that would compare the experiences of pregnant women with and without HIV who would take the drugs either periodically or monthly. It would need to recruit about seven hundred women. It would last up to two years. If it succeeded, it could make a lifesaving difference to millions of women and children across Africa.

Building that study, from the ground up, was Scott Filler's job.

———

Malawi, wedged against Tanzania and Zambia, is a narrow strip of land stretched along the shore of a narrow lake that separates it from Mozambique. It was an English colony once, the British Central African Protectorate. The English relinquished it in 1964, leaving its nine tribes a common language and a taste for heavy breakfasts of fried eggs and baked beans.

Scott's base in Malawi was Liwonde, a small town below the base of the lake on the Shire River, which runs down into Mozambique. Liwonde lies on a plain studded with baobab trees and abrupt, harsh ridges of dark spiked rock. It has one paved road. Where the road runs over the river at the south end of the town, there is a twenty-four-hour roadblock manned by soldiers carrying semiautomatic rifles. There is one hotel, a few guesthouses, a street market twice a week, and electricity for about six hours a day.

There is also a hospital, a good one by Malawian standards: the Machinga District Hospital, a cluster of wide, low brick buildings linked by dirt courtyards and surrounded by chain-link fence. About 380,000 people lived in Machinga district, on the east bank of the river. When they needed care, they went first to local health clinics, and then to the hospital if their problems were more serious. If they had money, nurses would care for them in one of the wards. Nurses provided almost all the care in the hospital. There were only a few doctors: one Malawian who was the hospital's director, and several volunteers from aid organizations.

If patients could not pay, they went to a second ward, where their families fed and tended them instead. During the day, family members were everywhere, squatting in the courtyards to tend small children or washing laundry by hand in open stone tubs along the hospital walls. In the evening, the families gathered to cook over open fires in one corner of the hospital grounds. Chickens and stray dogs wandered through the groups as they settled for the night.

In the opposite corner of the grounds was a dormitory for nursing students, a low brick building with a kitchen, a laundry, and a row of small bedrooms. At one end there was an office suite: two small rooms, a bathroom, and a closet with a lock. It was the office for Scott's project, and it was submerged in paper: stacks of blank mimeographed forms for enrolling patients in the study, keeping track of their visits, and recording their deliveries, and boxes of filled-out forms to be entered into a computer that he had hauled from Atlanta. The computer was also intended to give Scott email access; but it depended on phone lines, which on average worked every fourth day.

Getting the data into the computer was the responsibility of Leo Lesten, a slender twenty-three-year-old from the next district who had taken a computer course in South Africa. He lived in Liwonde with his eight- and twelve-year-old brothers. He had brought them to live with him after their father died; his mother, he said vaguely, was unable to care for them. The study also had a manager, Lloyd Chuckwawa; an accountant, Joyce Chilombo; two lab techs, Bulala and Scott Santula; a cleaning woman; and a driver. The clinical staff were four nurses hired for the study and two more on loan from the hospital. They were ruled over by a nursing supervisor: fifty-nine-year-old Catherine Malenga, whom everyone called "Ogogo," the Chichewa word for grandmother. Ogogo was a sturdy woman, barely five feet tall, who was kind to the patients but strict with the younger nurses. She wore her hair braided close to her scalp and twisted into a tiny topknot at the top of her head, and the crown-like arrangement reinforced her dignified air.

To entice women to participate in the study, Scott and his team had created their own prenatal care unit inside the hospital, which already had a mother and child clinic that operated every weekday morning. At about 8:00 a.m. every weekday, pregnant women and mothers with babies and toddlers squeezed onto benches in a light-filled square room at one end of the main hospital building. One by one, the hospital nurses who ran the clinic checked the women in, weighed them if they were pregnant or their babies if they were mothers, sorted them by problem and urgency, and sent them into the hallway to wait for another nurse to see them.

By 10:00 a.m., the big room would be empty and the benches and floor outside the examining rooms in the dark hall would be full of heavily pregnant women wrapped in two or three chitenjas, a sarong-like piece of printed cloth that served as an overskirt or a baby sling. In the dim light, the chitenjas made a brightly colored set of moving billboards. One bore an anti-AIDS message in French, another a Bible verse in Chichewa; two commemorated a national women's day, and one displayed a bad likeness of Michael Jackson set amidst guitars, microphones, and dollar symbols. Another was an ad for Coca-Cola, but washed so often the trademark red had faded to a thready frosted pink.

Almost all of the women were younger than twenty. They usually walked to the hospital, many of them from at least ten kilometers away. Once they reached the clinic, they might sit for hours. On most days there were two hundred or more women, and only one or two clinic nurses to treat them.

Scott's study had four nurses working every day. Every morning, one of them would wade into the crowds in the clinic's main room, winnow out girls who were pregnant for the first or second time—pregnancies when the loss of immunity would be most acute—and ask them to be screened for the study. If they were accepted, they would never again have to join the mob in the waiting room; they could come back to the study nurses for all the rest of their prenatal care. If they were not accepted, they would still get the same initial checkup, tests, and malaria pills as the women waiting to be seen in the clinic, without the wait. Women who were turned away were given a bar of laundry soap as a thank-you; women who were accepted, and returned for their next appointments, were reimbursed for their travel. If they stayed in the study until they delivered, they were given a baby-care kit—soap, a plastic basin, and a chitenja, items that their subsistence-farming families would not have the cash to buy.

The nurses were seldom turned down. "Women want to be in this study," Scott said. "After we've seen them, we give them a passbook to keep track of their appointments; they get that whether they join the study or not. We've seen women throw their passbooks away and try to enroll again, hoping they'll be chosen the second time."

The study's popularity was a lucky thing, because the task was huge. To finish with seven hundred study subjects, the staff would have to enroll many more, to compensate for women who would drop out. In addition, half of the participants had to be HIV-positive. The local rate of HIV infection was turning out to be almost 12 percent, instead of the 20 percent the malaria branch had predicted. That meant that, to secure his seven hundred participants, Scott and the staff would have to test and interview almost ten thousand women.

———

Workdays in Malawi began with a 7:30 a.m. meeting of the nursing staff; Ogogo always started with a prayer. They ended after dark and frequently in the dark, if the power had gone out again. Scott had gotten used to eating by paraffin lamp and typing in his hotel room while wearing a backpacking headlamp on an elastic band. He often worked late, because most nights it was too hot to sleep. The heat was made worse because protecting against mosquitoes demanded sleeping in long sleeves and long pants, and under a stifling bednet. The bednet had to be tucked beneath the mattress edges after you crawled under it, to make a barrier to the six-inch-long millipedes that also wanted to crawl inside.

It was a challenging assignment. There were only a handful of Caucasians in Liwonde and few people who spoke English as a first language. There had been cholera outbreaks the month before, a vivid demonstration of how unsafe the water was. Food was limited, because the country was still recovering from a famine in the dry season. The hotel restaurant's menu listed ten dishes, but on any one night there were only one or two to choose from. The basic food was nsima—white corn porridge, the local staple—augmented with a small portion of chicken, or chombo, a bony perch that was fished from the river and fried whole.

"It is hard to be here for any period of time," he said. "The work is great, it's very satisfying, but there are huge setbacks. I can sit down to look at the patient forms and find five errors in the first five I look at. It makes me wonder what errors occur while I'm gone."

Scott had spent two months in Malawi on the last trip and six weeks there on this one. He did not expect to return until September; his and Sami's baby was due in June. Sami was having a rough pregnancy. Increasingly he felt tugged back to Atlanta.

"I try to remember that every study client is someone's sister, someone's wife, and that their pregnancy has as much value to them as Sami's does to me," he said. "That's my link into this. It keeps me focused."

———

Inside the hospital, the study staff had two small rooms to work in. One served as a meeting room, spare examining room, and retreat for the nurses; it had a single metal cabinet that held all the patients' charts. The other was the study's lab, a tightly organized space only six feet wide that usually held six people at a time: both lab technicians, at least one nurse, several clients, and Lloyd, who entered the women's names into the study's ledgers and kept track of their appointments. Despite the crowd—the only safe place to sit was directly behind the door—it was calm compared to the chaos of bodies and babies in the clinic hallway outside.

Women who volunteered to be screened for the study were put through an elaborate series of tests and questions. They had to be at least sixteen years old, in their first or second pregnancies, pregnant for at least sixteen weeks but no more than twenty-eight weeks, and willing to be tested for HIV and syphilis. All the women who were HIV-positive were enrolled in the study; a random choice from the negatives was enrolled to balance each positive.

On a brilliantly clear morning in mid-March, three young women filed into the lab to have their blood drawn for testing. They had already agreed to HIV testing and been given physicals by the nurses. They were the 602nd, 603rd, and 604th patients screened by the study; their names were Dorothy, Lucy, and Emmie.

Dorothy was sixteen years old and pregnant for the first time. She smiled and hid her face in her hands when Ogogo asked her whether she had felt the baby move. Lucy was seventeen. Emmie was twenty, married to a car mechanic, and had a three-year-old child. She had a charming gap between her front teeth and the broad cheekbones of the Yao tribal group; when Santula bent over her arm to draw blood, she spoke to him in Yao.

"She said people told her not to come to the hospital, because they are stealing blood there," he said. "She said she told them she would go see for herself."

For several months, southern Malawi had been plagued by rumors that vampires were creeping into huts late at night to steal blood from villagers. The vampires were employed by the government, the rumors said; the government had traded the blood to international aid agencies in exchange for food. It seemed farcical, but the results were sobering. A Malawian man had been stoned to death by a mob that accused him of colluding with the vampires, and three foreign priests had been attacked and badly bruised.

The rumors had not yet touched Scott's study. The staff seemed unconcerned.

"There are a lot of misconceptions," Lloyd said. "Some say if you take blood from someone, they will die. Others say we are taking the blood to sell to the mzungus, the white people. But some, they understand."

To test the girls' HIV status, the lab techs used European rapid tests that returned results within fifteen minutes. Santula lined up the tests on the lab counter, two for each girl, and dripped blood carefully onto them from pipettes. Dorothy and Emmie went to other rooms in the clinic to get vaccinations and give stool and urine samples. Lucy was feverish with an attack of malaria; she curled up in a corner of the floor to rest.

Santula checked the test strips. Two sets were blank. One was positive. It was Emmie's. Ogogo took her into the other room to deliver the news.

Neither of the others joined the study. Lloyd gave them bars of laundry soap to say thank you. They left for the long walks home.

The last thing the study team did every day was to drive the new participants home. It was partly a courtesy—the screening lasted so long that the regular clinic was empty by the time the study finished enrolling girls for the day—but mostly strategic. To give the women antimalarials and keep gathering data on them, the study needed the participants to come back to the hospital once a month. If they did not, the staff went out to find them. The last thing folded into each new patient's chart was a Polaroid of her face and a hand-drawn map of the route to her house.

It could be a complicated trip. Once off the paved road, navigating in Liwonde meant taking an off-road vehicle up dirt roads that progressively narrowed to single tracks overgrown with waist-high grass and then to walking trails. The paths wound through corn that was more than seven feet high. It was impossible to see more than two or three feet ahead. Villages were audible long before they came into view between the corn stalks. The paths ended abruptly in beaten-earth courtyards full of children and goats.

Emmie lived more than fifteen kilometers from the hospital on a foothill of Mount Mulangi, the biggest feature on the horizon south of Liwonde. The route passed a mosque, fields of tobacco, a pump, and a hut with a sign identifying it as the local Adventist church. Her village was a family cluster of fifteen huts set in a packed-earth clearing dotted with beds of bougainvillea. Rabbits, let out of a primitive hutch for the day, nibbled at the flowers.

Most of the group's men were absent. Emmie's sister-in-law, a slender woman in her thirties with a scar on one cheek, welcomed the visitors, putting them on chairs made of scavenged building materials. Diana Chinansi, one of the study nurses, explained that Emmie had joined the study and would have to return to the hospital every month.

Nothing was said about her diagnosis. There seemed little point: Anti-AIDS drugs are not available in Malawi. If Emmie stayed with the study and delivered her baby at the hospital, the staff would give her a single dose of nevirapine to prevent HIV from passing to her child. That was all that could be done.

Emmie's ultimate fate was cruelly obvious: She was unlikely to live more than a few years. But in the short term, it was unclear what her diagnosis would mean to her life. Many women did not tell their spouses, Ogogo said. Sometimes it was out of knowledge that the husband was the source of the infection. Sometimes it was simply fear of what he would do.

"Some men will ask for a divorce," she said. "Some will go to another woman. But some will forgive each other. Malawian women are very strong. They go on."

AIDS was not spoken of much in Malawi, but its effects were everywhere. Half a kilometer south of the hospital stood a broad painted sign: New Style Coffin Workshop. The business—a mud-brick house and a row of open sheds strung along the edge of the road to Zomba, the next town—belonged to German Kaunde, a short, strong man in his sixties. Kaunde wore secondhand dress slacks, red rubber flip-flops, and the white cap of an observant Moslem. His two front teeth were missing.

Kaunde had started out making furniture in 1962—doors, chairs, tables, and beds. Business had been good, but in the 1980s it dropped off, and people started asking him to make coffins. In 1989, he had switched to making coffins only.

It had been a good business. Most of Kaunde's seven children worked with him, along with four young men from the area. In most weeks, they sold five or six coffins. Each one took a day to make, and cost up to a month's wages to buy. But the business was growing less profitable—not because fewer people were dying, but because so many other coffin builders had opened. To compete, he and his sons had branched out, opening coffin shops in three other towns. The new businesses—one was twenty kilometers away—were doing well. To visit their shops, Kaunde and his sons rode the overcrowded minibuses that plied the paved roads, clinging to the roof racks when the seats were full.

He did not know why so many people wanted coffins, Kaunde said. It was not his business to know. People wanted coffins; he made them, and people bought them, and that was good enough. He made the same gesture the study staff had made, the shrug of discomfort, the shifting of the eyes to some spot in the distance. Even amidst the evidence of its impact—the pale chips of wood underfoot from beveling the coffin lids, the ringing of a hammer shaping a metal handle—AIDS was too taboo to be discussed.

"HIV is always in your face here," Scott said. "In the past month, three members of the hospital staff have had family die of it. My biggest fear is that one of our people will die."

———

For Scott's study to succeed, it was crucial to follow the women all the way to delivery, and the delivery had to be in the hospital. Only there could the researchers gather the blood and tissue samples that would prove which regimen did a better job of protecting against malaria. The blood samples had to be taken within forty-eight hours of birth, and the placenta needed to be biopsied quickly. If a woman gave birth in her village, she would never get to the hospital in time. Without the sample results, details about her could not be used in the study. Her months of trekking to the hospital, and the staff's work to take care of her, would be for nothing.

Most women, though, gave birth at home, with the help of a traditional birth attendant—not a Western-style midwife, but a village woman who had been trained by an older woman and might know some herbal medicine as well. The attendants were controversial, not just in Malawi but throughout Southern Africa. Governments wanted women to deliver in hospitals, not at home without medical care or access to the drugs that would prevent HIV transmission from mother to baby.

It was a complex problem. Few women could face walking five kilometers in active labor and then waiting for a crowded minibus, which might take a half a day to come, to get them the rest of the way to the hospital. The answer was to get the women to the hospital well in advance of delivery, so several governments including Malawi's had begun building hostels that would house women for the last month of pregnancy. But removing a woman for several weeks from a subsistence-farming family took away a key laborer, the sole source of child care and probably the only preparer of food.

For Scott, the solution to those issues was to compensate the study participants coming to Liwonde's hostel, Guardian House, not with money but with baby-care kits and clothing for the women and bags of nsima for their families. Dealing with the birth attendants was more complicated. The women earned a living caring for pregnant women and newborns. As important as the income was the status and influence that went with the job. If women began delivering in hospitals, the attendants would lose both their livelihood and their position. And given the tight, tiny societies of the villages, extended family groups that might hold fewer than thirty relatives, few women would go to the hospital to deliver unless the local birth attendant indicated that she approved.

Scott and Ogogo had developed what they hoped was a plan. If a birth attendant's client delivered at the hospital, the study would pay the attendant as much money as if she had delivered the baby herself. They floated the idea at a meeting in mid-March with twenty-four attendants from the Machinga district. The women had drifted in on foot, curtseying to Scott, perching briefly on the hospital's hard-backed chairs, and then slipping out of them to sit straight-legged on the floor.

They chatted animatedly among themselves, accepted snacks of cookies and Fanta, and sang call-and-response songs, clapping and laughing. But when Scott described his proposal, and Ogogo translated it, they were silent.

Scott was frustrated. "I look at my notes from November, and they say, 'birth-attendant issue?' and then I look at notes I made last week, and they say the same thing," he said. "This is so important for women's health, and it's critical for the study. Every woman who delivers outside the hospital means this study goes another day."

Scott's concerns went beyond gathering data. He was accustomed to taking care of patients, and in Liwonde he was surrounded by them. Both wards of the hospital were full of men and women in the desperate last stages of AIDS and TB. Under normal circumstances he would have waded in, but he could not risk acquiring something that would pose a risk to Sami or their child.

Sami was always on Scott's mind. He was thousands of miles away from her, and unable to email her or to talk to her for more than a few minutes every few days. He had to trust that their family and friends would take care of her. But he could take care of Liwonde's pregnant women, if the birth attendants would cooperate.

It was not solely a question of a Western doctor believing he knew better. Delivering a baby in a village was objectively risky: Across Africa, more than one woman in two hundred died every year from labor complications, infection, or bleeding after delivery. Malarial anemia made the bleeding worse. And pregnant women in Malawi sometimes put themselves further at risk, taking a traditional medicine to bring on labor in hopes of getting the delivery over quickly. Every week, Machinga hospital surgeons performed emergency Cesareans and hysterectomies on women whose uteruses had ruptured under the pressure of the herb-induced contractions. A woman whose uterus ruptured in the bush would have no chance of survival at all.

If the birth attendants would not listen to the study team, perhaps they would pay attention to one of their own. On a blazing Saturday morning when no regular clinic was scheduled, Scott and Ogogo set off to visit a powerful local woman named Funny Kachingwe, who ran her own clinic and delivered several dozen babies a month.

They had been warned it was not an easy place to find. The route started with a ten-kilometer drive on the paved road north of Liwonde, followed by a left turn into high grass and a two-kilometer drive up a narrow track between fields of corn. That was as far as the Jeep could go. It took an hour's hike to reach Kachingwe's house: up hills, between corn fields, across two rice paddies, and through a shallow, rapid stream more than twenty feet across.

Kachingwe—her clients called her "Mai," Chichewa for mother—was a tall, light-skinned woman with broad shoulders and wide hips. She showed off her settlement with pride: a white-washed stucco house with a porch and a metal roof; a shoulder-high dovecote woven out of twigs for pigeons, and a long, low brick building for chickens and goats; and the "hospital," five mud-brick huts roofed with reeds. One hut was an examining room; one was a pharmacy, filled from wall to wall with stacks of roots and leaves for traditional medicine; one was the clinic, where people who needed several days of treatment stayed overnight. The hospital was popular: More than twenty clients sat against the hut walls, out of the brutal sun.

Set off to the side behind a low wall were the two remaining huts, much smaller than the rest. They were the obstetrics ward. In one, two women who had given birth the previous evening nursed their newborns, while two others in the early stages of labor waited for something to happen. In the other—a small square box without windows, hot and dark—a woman lay by herself on a dried-grass mat, breathing hard between contractions, very close to giving birth.

Mai unrolled mats on the ground near the dovecote, under a tree but out of reach of a tethered goat that nibbled on the tires of a bicycle propped against the trunk. From the house, she brought a three-ring binder filled with mimeographed log pages, a gift from a government nurse appointed by the district to keep track of the local birth attendants. The nurse was supposed to come every month, though Mai had not seen the woman for twelve weeks. But she had completed the log regardless. Its columns were carefully filled out: Fifteen clients in the first eight days of March. All fifteen of the babies had lived. Six of the mothers had died.

At the corner of the obstetrics hut, one of Mai's assistants beckoned:

The baby was on its way. Mai and Ogogo bustled to their feet. Scott stayed behind, sitting on a sawed-off piece of tree trunk. He reached for the log. A white chicken stepped carefully around the tree roots, followed by five small striped chicks.

"This is terrible," he said. He looked around at the mud-brick hospital and the hut where his chief nurse had disappeared. "It's appalling. No woman should ever have to deliver a baby this way." He tossed the log book back on the mat.

After forty-five minutes, Ogogo appeared around the corner, walking quickly, smiling and clapping her hands. "The mother is fine," she said. "The baby is fine."

She reached the edge of the mat and looked down. "It is a baby boy," she said. "Shall we name him Scott?"

———

When Scott was in Liwonde, he met with the study staff twice a day. On his last day there in March, Diana arrived late to the morning gathering. She had been working since the night before in the hospital's delivery ward.

It had been a bad night, she said. A woman pregnant with twins had been brought in by ambulance with meningitis; she was unconscious, and the high fever had sent her into premature labor. One twin had died. The other had lived, saved by an emergency C-section. But in the middle of the C-section, the power had failed again, shutting off the ventilator. There was no fuel in the hospital's generator, so the surgeon had finished the operation by paraffin lamp while the nurses inflated the mother's lungs by hand. The mother might survive, Diana said. It seemed unlikely that the baby would.

But there was good news, Ogogo added: One of the study's first participants, patient 128, had come in from her village to give birth in the hospital. In one day, eleven women enrolled earlier in the study had returned for their monthly appointments. And one, according to her chart, had made four visits so far to the study, with one still to go.

Scott was thrilled. He was leaving after the meeting for the several-hour drive to Blantyre, the nearest town with an airport. The next day, he would start the thirty hours of flights that would bring him to Johannesburg, Cape Town, and then home. With Ogogo's report, he felt more confident that the study would succeed while he was gone.

"There has never been a study that got patients beyond three doses, and this woman might get to five," he said. "Of course, we don't know yet if the monthly regimen confers any benefit. But this way, we'll know."

TEN

Tuberculosis

1999–2000, Baltimore
and New York

IT WAS BARELY 5:00 A.M., and chilly for spring, but the Brooklyn YMCA was bustling. Handmade posters pointed the way to a gym where a buzz was already building. Young men and a few women, African-American and Latino, stood patiently in a line that snaked up to a cafeteria table where volunteers were selling tickets and writing down names. Past the table, ticket-holders headed for the locker rooms, hoisting backpacks stuffed with shoes and hair dryers and hanger bags whose half-open zippers spilled out slinky dresses and tightly tailored suits.

In less than an hour, the men disappearing into the locker rooms would burst out into the gym, striding and twirling down a makeshift runway, transformed by effort and attitude into near-perfect facsimiles of models, movie stars, and TV characters. The biggest vogue ball of the winter—an underground twelve-hour event that had lured transsexual and cross-dressing men to New York from as far south as Atlanta—was about to get under way.

173

Off to the side of the hallway, CDC researchers Peter McElroy and Renee Ridzon watched the growing crowd with fascination fogged over by lack of sleep. They had worked for months to identify and infiltrate the tightly knit, seldom-disclosed relationships binding together hundreds of men who preferred to appear in public as women. They had attended a small ball in Baltimore weeks earlier, and some of the friends they made there had urged them to come to New York. Their new acquaintances implied that until they saw a full-scale ball, a concentrated combination of elegance, bitchery, and aspirational yearning, they would miss an essential element of the community they needed to understand.

In the crowd in the hallway, a young woman waved at McElroy. Puzzled—he was sure he did not know this longhaired, carefully made-up vision in pressed jeans and high heels—he left Ridzon and walked over to her. She smiled as he came closer.

"You don't remember me, do you?" she asked.

Suddenly, he did. He recognized the voice, though nothing else. When they had met for lunch six months earlier, she had been a he.

———

McElroy, a Ph.D. in epidemiology, and Ridzon, an infectious disease physician, had come to Brooklyn in pursuit of one of the oldest plagues to affect mankind, and one of the most fiercely resurgent: tuberculosis.

Evidence of the lung-destroying disease predates the alphabet. Signs of infection have been found in Egyptian mummies. TB and humans co-existed for millennia, until the enormous social changes triggered by the Industrial Revolution changed the balance between man and disease. Across Europe, rural residents accustomed to clean living and a moderate level of nutrition flooded into the crowded new slums of cities. Packed close together, working long hours and unable to afford decent food, they were virgin soil for TB to flourish in. By the nineteenth century, one out of every ten Europeans died of TB.

The disease was so commonplace that it altered concepts of art and beauty. The relative youth of its frequently famous victims—John

Keats, Frederic Chopin, all three of the Brontë sisters, Anton Chekhov, and D. H. Lawrence—made the infection paradoxically desirable. Authors and opera composers gave the disease to their romantic heroines, creating irresistible popular symbols of seduction, tragedy, and decay. Advanced TB destroys lung tissue, starving the body of oxygen. Its outward signs—pale skin, wasted muscles, fatigue, and a feverish flush—became morbidly fashionable, a nineteenth-century version of heroin chic.

The organism responsible for the disease, *Mycobacterium tuberculosis,* was identified by Robert Koch in 1882. X-rays, developed thirteen years later, allowed doctors to see the damage it did to the lungs and understand how far a case of the disease had progressed. The first drug that was successful against the organism, streptomycin, was released in 1944. It was followed by the rest of the first-line drugs used against TB: isoniazid and pyrazinamide, developed in the 1950s, and ethambutol and rifampin, developed in the 1960s. By the 1970s, the rate of active cases of TB fell dramatically.

"In residency, I hardly saw any patients with tuberculosis," said Ridzon, who entered medical school in St. Louis in 1982. "Once in a while one would come along, and the attending physicians would say, 'That's TB. You won't ever have to deal with that—it's going away.'"

By the mid-1980s, it roared back. Treatment had been so successful that big cities, where most cases were concentrated, rerouted clinic and treatment funds to other diseases, especially newly identified HIV, which was making punishing demands on public health. The decisions to redirect scarce funds made sense at the time. Viewed through the lenses of TB biology and the demands of treating the disease, though, they were deeply shortsighted. One out of every ten people infected with TB develops active TB disease. If they are not treated, they can infect an average of ten more people in a year. Successfully treating active TB requires taking a cocktail of several of the five first-line drugs for at least six months, a program that few people can follow unless a health worker coaches or nags them through it. The remaining nine infected people do not pass on the disease; they develop latent infections, in which the bacteria remain in the body but are kept under control by the immune system. One in ten of them, though, will develop active TB and become contagious later in life, when age or another infection undermines immunity. Eliminating latent TB infection requires at least two months of treatment with at least one of the first-line drugs.

There were other factors contributing to the resurgent epidemic. The first was HIV. Its assault on the immune system changes the mathematics of TB. When HIV-positive people become infected with the bacteria, two out of five of them—four times as many as in healthy people—develop full-blown tuberculosis. And when someone with a latent TB infection becomes HIV-infected, the chance that they will progress to active disease rises from 10 percent in their lifetime to 10 percent per year.

The second contributing factor was a by-product of health agencies' inattention to TB. Active cases were still detected and given the drugs needed to control the disease, and many of the patients started on the lengthy course of drugs. But, left to themselves, few of the infected managed to finish the regimens. It was a situation tailor-made for the Darwinian emergence of TB strains that were resistant to at least one, and sometimes two, of the first-line drugs. In 1991, the CDC compared national statistics on resistant cases with a survey it had completed five years earlier. In 1991, 14.4 percent of TB infections were resistant to one drug; 3.1 percent were resistant to the two most important drugs, isoniazid and rifampin. In 1986, the percentage of infections resistant to those two drugs had been only 0.5 percent, one-sixth of the 1991 rate.

The development of multidrug-resistant TB posed two major problems. The first was a severe exacerbation of the difficulty of treatment. Drug regimens for multidrug-resistant TB, usually abbreviated as MDR TB, take three to four times as long to complete, up to twenty-four months, and cure only 60 percent of patients instead of close to 100 percent. The second was that MDR TB was not occurring randomly; it was beginning to cluster. Between 1990 and 1992, the CDC uncovered seven outbreaks in hospitals and a prison in Florida and New York that collectively included more than two hundred patients. Almost all of the patients had HIV, and almost all were infected with TB strains that were resistant to both isoniazid and rifampin. Some harbored strains that resisted all five first-line drugs and two of the second-line, less effective drugs as well. The outbreaks were ferocious: Between 70 and 90 percent of the infected patients and inmates died. And they were hard to contain: Nine hospital workers and prison guards also developed the disease, and five of them died too.

By 1993, resurgent TB had become such a crisis that the World Health Organization, for the first time in its history, declared a global health emergency. In 1997, a WHO survey of thirty-five countries found that at least one-third of them had at least 1,000 patients with MDR TB. In Latvia, 22 percent of all TB patients had strains resisting at least the two main drugs; in the Dominican Republic, 9 percent; in Russia, 7 percent. In America, drug-resistant TB had been found in forty-two states. In 1999, there were 8.4 million new cases of TB worldwide.

In August 1999, the Baltimore City Health Department discovered thirteen cases of tuberculosis among young African-American men, eight of them HIV-positive. The health department called the CDC for help. Peter McElroy, three weeks out of EIS training, took the call.

———

McElroy, who was thirty-five when he came to the EIS, had suspected his work might lead him in some unexpected directions. In 1999, the year he joined, the overall U.S. epidemic was coming under control again, but there were troubling trends that signaled TB would become harder to handle. More and more, the disease was coming into the country via visitors and legal and illegal immigrants. In 1999, 44 percent of all U.S. cases of TB were among those born outside the country. The cases among native-born Americans were increasingly clustered in small pockets of the disenfranchised: low-income families, homeless people, the incarcerated, and the invisible members of the all-cash economy—drug users, sex workers, and undocumented aliens.

In other words, the easy cases were already taken care of. Finding and treating the remaining ones required a different set of tools than the traditional public-health epidemiology—diagnose the case, ask about the infectious person's social contacts, test and treat the contacts—that TB-control programs had relied on for a century. Just like the traditional cases, which were connected by family, school, or business relationships, the new outbreaks were linked, but in ways hidden from mainstream society. Being a TB detective in the late 1990s meant learning to map an unfamiliar landscape.

McElroy was accustomed to working in unusual locations. As a University of Michigan graduate student, he had been a Peace Corps volunteer in Kenya. He had gone back almost ten years later to do dissertation research on malarial anemia in children. Despite that international background, he had asked when he joined the EIS not to be assigned to a job that would send him abroad. He wanted the experience of working inside a well-developed public health system. He chose to go into TB because it had such a system, assembled by local, state, and national health authorities over more than one hundred years. He expected to be working on small outbreaks, and he knew enough about the changing distribution of the disease to expect them to be challenging.

He had no idea. TB took the researcher into a filthy squat in a poor neighborhood of St. Louis to interview a woman who shared the same multiple-drug-resistant strain as nine other people. It also took him into the back rooms of strip clubs in Wichita. Over seven years, ten men, nine women, and three children had come down with TB there; the most obvious link was that seven of the nine women were exotic dancers. (Most of the adult cases were also crack users who shared the drug by shotgunning, breathing the smoke into each other's mouths. When the cluster was analyzed, drug use proved to be a stronger link between the cases.)

It took him, eventually, to Raleigh, North Carolina—and to being forced to kneel in the street, with his hands behind his head and his forehead on the bumper of his car, while seven police officers trained their guns on him.

McElroy and a helper, a Raleigh municipal employee, had been looking for a resident of the local homeless shelter, a man with suspected TB who needed to be put on a drug treatment program to protect him from infecting others. The shelter, a converted warehouse that held more than 350 men, harbored an explosive outbreak: twenty-five cases of active TB and another 119 cases of latent infection who needed treatment to prevent them from progressing to full-blown disease.

It was late afternoon, and the shelter had turned its overnight guests out for the day. The homeless population in Raleigh was moderately transient; men tended to stay there for only a few weeks before moving farther up or down the East Coast. McElroy feared that the suspected patient might have headed out of town, but there was a chance that he was merely lingering in the neighborhood until the shelter opened again for the night. The epidemiologist and the city employee, who worked at the shelter, had set out to look for him. After several blocks, a police car pulled up behind them.

"They pulled us over, but the officer stayed in his car, while I sat there wondering what the heck was going on," McElroy said. "Then five minutes later six other cars all converged behind us, and the officers started shouting at me to throw my keys out of the window and then get out of the car with my hands behind my head and back up to the back of the vehicle. I kept trying to peek behind me, and every time I did, they were pointing the guns right at us."

The police patted down McElroy and his passenger, and put them in the back of separate squad cars. One of them started asking McElroy what he was doing on the street he had been driving down. Two others began searching the car he had been forced to abandon.

"I said I didn't know which street it was, I just knew that we had just come from the city shelter a few streets away," he said. "I identified myself three times, the first time while there was a gun at my head, but it didn't seem to make a difference."

After forty-five minutes, McElroy and his helper were released. Furious, he drove after the police to their station downtown, where the desk commander explained that their car had been mistaken for one spotted earlier in the day in a drug deal. He declined to apologize. The implication, never spelled out but clear nonetheless, was that the city employee, a black man, was the drug dealer; McElroy, blond and blue-eyed, his customer.

It made sense, the epidemiologist thought later, that some of the vulnerable people he had been looking for tried so hard to keep their existence invisible. No wonder they were so disinclined to trust him when he tracked them down to ask where and with whom they spent their time. "It really gave me an appreciation for what some people in this country have to put up with," he said. He had spent significant time in one of the most unpredictable countries in Africa, but the lone time he was abused by authorities was after he came home.

————

Public health officials in Baltimore knew from the start that there was something anomalous about their outbreak. The cases were all young; that was unusual. And twelve of the thirteen were visibly transgender. Some had appeared at the health department dressed as women, while others had long hair or long painted nails, suggesting that they dressed in drag some days of their lives. Some of them took feminizing hormones, but they were not transsexuals as they defined the term. Few of them planned on becoming surgically female. Despite their clothes and grooming, they saw themselves as men who liked to have sex with men.

Baltimore knew the cases were an outbreak because, unlike most health departments, it performed DNA fingerprinting on every TB isolate collected from a suspected patient. The patterns generated by the bacteria taken from the young men were identical. They all had the same strain of TB, and they had all acquired it recently. The mystery was how the outbreak had happened, and how far it had gone.

For McElroy, the group was a perfect example of the hidden relationships by which TB spread. When they were interviewed, the young men all said that they belonged to a "house," a self-constructed family with a mother and sometimes a father, both men. House members seldom lived in the same place, but they hung out together and took care of each other. A few of them had low-level jobs. Most managed by hustling or stealing. Several turned tricks.

"They had been completely ostracized by their families, so they stuck close together," McElroy said. "They were out on the streets all night, into the early morning. There was a lot of drug use and a lot of needle sharing going on, though the needle sharing was not so much for illegal drugs as for black market estrogen and silicone. Between the needles, the drug use, and the commercial sex, their HIV risk was higher than any group you could imagine."

The close relationships in the house explained how the Baltimore men could have infected each other: TB, an airborne disease, spreads easily in close quarters. But they also suggested that the outbreak reached beyond the city. For this section of the transgender world, houses were a fundamental social unit. There were several dozen up and down the East Coast, centered in New York but reaching north and south of the city. Houses put on balls where members displayed their finesse at dressing up in dozens of styles, from elegant evening wear to perfect imitations of businessmen, school kids, and military officers. The most prestigious balls were in New York, and members of the Baltimore clan traveled there frequently.

The researchers were unnerved. If the infected men in Baltimore had gone to New York, it was likely they had either acquired TB there, or taken it with them and passed it on. McElroy and Ridzon needed to find the men that their Baltimore patients had partied with in New York City. But few of the house members knew each other's real names.

"The houses have a house name—you drop your birth name and use that," Ridzon said. "Some of the guys did drag shows and had performance names for those. They were all known to each other by pseudonyms—or someone would say, 'I don't remember her name, but she had her cheeks done.'"

And unlike Baltimore, New York City did not at the time do DNA fingerprinting on its TB cases. The testing was prohibitively expensive because New York had thousands of patients every year. But genotyping was essential for the investigators to confirm the possible connections between New York and Baltimore. There was no other way to tell whether the New York cases shared the same strain as the Baltimore outbreak.

To find out whom they should test, the investigators fell back on shoe-leather epidemiology. They went to New York, checked in at TB clinics around the city, and asked the staff to pull the medical charts for any patients who matched the demographics of the Baltimore outbreak: HIV-positive African-American men in their early twenties. Then they read the charts themselves. There were a lot of charts: Every cluster of cases in New York included young black men made vulnerable to the disease by HIV infection.

"Chart after chart would have statements in it like, 'Patient travels to Baltimore'; 'Patient unable to receive therapy today because he's in Baltimore,'" McElroy said. "Sometimes the nurses had written additional comments: 'Patient comes in periodically dressed as a woman'; 'Patient has long fingernails and wears lipstick.'"

The details in the charts had been unimportant to the New York clinics. No one there knew about the Baltimore outbreak. In the staff's view, as long as patients showed up for their appointments, the other places they went were irrelevant. And no one had thought to ask about the obvious lifestyle clues. There was no reason to, since TB is not a sexually transmitted disease.

Armed with those details, McElroy and Ridzon asked the clinics to pull from their freezers whatever bacterial isolates remained from the patients, and send them to the CDC for analysis. Out of the first thirty patients they checked, seven matched the Baltimore TB strain. They did the same for Philadelphia, Newark, and Washington, D.C. And they ran the molecular fingerprint through a new TB database at the CDC that held genotypes from five states—Arkansas, Maryland, Massachusetts, Michigan, and New Jersey—as well as five counties in Texas, and greater San Francisco. Simultaneously—because, thanks to the medical charts, they now had the patients' real names and last known address—the New York health department plugged information on the newly found cases with the Baltimore strain of bacteria into a computer program. It cross-matched their addresses against the rest of the TB patients in New York.

The genotyping and the address check more than doubled the size of the outbreak. There were not eighteen patients, but thirty-nine, distributed across Maryland, New Jersey, and New York. Thirty were men; thirty-six were black; nineteen of them belonged to the same house. The outbreak had spread beyond their tight-knit community, though. Three of the women were family and co-workers of one of the New Jersey patients. A Maryland woman had been a custodian at a hospital where a patient had been treated. A woman in Baltimore was friendly with the owners of a nightclub where some of that city's patients hung out. And in New York, a one-year-old with the Baltimore strain of TB lived across the hall from the apartment of one of the transgender patients, though neither the patient nor the baby's mother could remember any contact between them.

The work the researchers had done had defined the outbreak for them, but those findings were not enough. They still did not know the locations where the disease was being transmitted, and they had no reason to believe that transmission had stopped. To answer their questions, they needed to go deeper into the transgender world.

———

Preventing the fast-moving disease from causing more cases of tuberculosis was crucial, because the group in which it was spreading was so vulnerable. At least twenty-one of the thirty-nine patients were HIV-infected. By the time McElroy and Ridzon arrived in New York, three were dead.

"The fatality rate in this cluster of cases was higher than any others I have investigated, extraordinarily high," McElroy said. "Hardly any of these guys were on antiretroviral therapy. Most of them didn't know they were positive—they were diagnosed with HIV at the same time they found they had TB."

The child's case was especially troubling. The traditional understanding of TB dictated that close, prolonged contact was necessary for infection, but if the child had had any contact with the patient who lived across the hall, it had been brief and fleeting. It made the investigators worry that this TB strain might be different.

That raised a fresh set of fears. The patients they had interviewed had told them about the transgender balls. Within the community, the gatherings were such a source of affirmation and glory that men made extraordinary efforts to be there, even when they had to travel all night by bus or jam into a crowded apartment to crash for a few hours on the floor. If this strain of the disease could be passed by casual contact, then the balls might be a serious health hazard for anyone who attended. But if the investigators charged in to demand that the competitions be closed, they would drive the gatherings further underground and lose the opportunity to halt the continuing outbreak.

Seeking a better understanding of the community, and hoping to find a little leverage, McElroy and Ridzon set out to understand the transgendered life. They discovered it was wider and better organized, and more fragmented, than they imagined.

"I thought this was a marginalized, unknown population," said Ridzon, who had been an EIS officer seven years before McElroy and stayed to work with the CDC's TB division. "But when I got into it, I discovered there were websites, and magazines, and a coherent culture that I knew nothing about."

Which may mean that work at the CDC kept its researchers too busy to pay much attention to pop culture. By 1999, transvestites had passed their fifteenth minute of fame and drag had lost most of its power to shock. The award-winning documentary *Paris Is Burning,* which recorded the balls of Harlem, was released in 1990; so was the Madonna video "Vogue," which brought the style into the mainstream. Nine years later, Lypsinka—the performance persona of entertainer John Epperson—had not only had a show on Broadway but had done a Gap ad. Drag diva RuPaul, whose real name was Andre Charles, had scored a No. 1 single and been the "face" of a major makeup line, and was hosting a six-day-a-week talk show on VH-1.

Nevertheless, the world of the balls—black, urban, low-income— remained tightly closed even to other transgendered men.

"We started to understand that saying 'the transgender community' was like saying 'the heterosexual community,' that's how diverse it was," McElroy said. "We were looking for young African-American men, and we met white businessmen and Latino women. One person we talked to was a former gunnery sergeant in the Marines who had been married but realized he was not comfortable with his gender identity. By the time we met, he was a postoperative transsexual, a middle-aged white woman. She didn't know any more about the ball scene than we did."

The researchers began to realize why the balls were still so underground. Socially, the participants had two strikes against them: They were minorities and they were gay. Middle-class America might find drag queens amusing and glamorous, but these men lived in cultures—African-American and Latino home life, and the street life of New York City—where manliness was still traditionally defined.

The balls' closed society made it imperative for Ridzon and McElroy to recruit an ambassador, someone from within the community who would agree to be their guide. They found him in Baltimore: one of the outbreak patients, who liked talking to them. Over weeks, as the three went out for lunch, he drew a detailed portrait of the intense loyalty and fierce rivalries that came with house membership, the need to be fabulous, the drive to be "legendary"—the highest accolade the community could bestow. He recited the names of the best-known houses: the House of Chanel, the House of St. Laurent; Ninja, La Mer, Adonis, Xtravaganza; La Beija, whose matriarch Pepper had starred in *Paris Is Burning*.

Their informant was nineteen years old. Before the TB diagnosis, he had been taking black-market estrogen to give him curves and take away his facial hair. Estrogen, though, dilutes the effectiveness of rifampin, one of the most-used drugs for TB.

"She got it," Ridzon said. "She understood that she wasn't going to buck the disease, so for six months she gave up the estrogen. She cut her hair, and cut off her nails; by the time we met her, she looked androgynous."

By the time the team had gone on to New York, their friend had finished the mandatory six months of TB treatment, started back on hormones, and reclaimed his female identity. By the time she waved to McElroy in the YMCA hallway, she had long hair, long nails, soft skin, and breasts.

"She was beautiful," McElroy said. "I would never have known her."

————

Their guide made it clear that, to understand the ball culture, they had to go to the gatherings.

"And he was right," McElroy said. "How could I ever claim to know the dynamics of TB transmission in this cluster of cases without seeing firsthand exactly what their life involves?"

There was another reason to go. The society of the houses was a rigid meritocracy whose essential currency was respect. Men emerged as candidates for house leaders because they displayed an edgy stylishness that made them stand out. They confirmed their status as mothers when they won more prizes at the balls than anyone else. To communicate the community's peril, and to see enough of ball society to understand where TB was being transmitted, McElroy and Ridzon had to get the mothers on the researchers' side.

None of the patients in the Baltimore outbreak were mothers.

"Leaders of that community have a lot of power and influence," McElroy said. "They're the guys that the younger transgender kids look up to. And to them, because they're so used to being picked on by society, we looked like just another authority coming in to bash them. So attending the balls was a way to get to the influential people and make sure we weren't alienating them."

It was also a chance to warn the community leaders about an underappreciated threat. Based on the patients they had identified and the case histories they had heard from TB clinic staff, the investigators thought the houses were likely to have a high rate of HIV infection. "Throw TB into the mix, and it becomes a disaster," McElroy said. "There is no known risk factor that promotes progression to active TB disease faster than HIV infection does."

The investigators visited several balls in Baltimore, and then the big one in New York. They came away dazzled by the glamour of the gatherings and moved by their intensity. They also emerged convinced that the balls were not the places where TB was being transmitted. They had feared the settings would resemble a nightclub, with low ceilings and no ventilation, a place where the lack of air circulation would allow bacteria to travel easily between people. But the balls turned out to be held in gyms and rental halls, high-ceilinged open places with roaring ventilation systems.

It was more likely, they realized, that the men had caught the disease on the way to and from the balls, in the overcrowded apartments where they would stay for several days. Or longer, as it turned out.

"A lot of the patients were essentially homeless, but not in the traditional sense of living in shelters," McElroy said. "They were sofa-surfing, going from apartment to apartment for periods of time. When we asked about the months preceding their diagnosis, without exception, everybody had stayed in the apartment of another person who had TB."

That recognition shut down the outbreak, for the most part. The cases and their contacts were treated by city clinics. Most completed their TB treatment and went on with their lives, though two-thirds of them were left with the new knowledge that they were HIV-positive and had few resources to pay for treatment. By 2001, six of the patients had died.

There remained, though, one group of cases that McElroy and Ridzon could not explain. Three of the outbreak patients in Baltimore were middle-aged married men. They were not in the transgender lifestyle; they were not even cross-dressers. They swore they had not spent any time with transvestites; as far as they knew, they had never met one.

Though they could not prove it, the investigators suspected that the men knew one or two transvestites very well.

"Because of the way they dressed, the young African-American transgender kids had a hard time finding employment," McElroy said. "So commercial sex work was a big part of their lives. The ones who would show up at the balls dressed so beautifully might a few hours earlier have been turning tricks on the street or in a bar.

"We're pretty sure that's where the heterosexual guys got infected, in a pick-up bar where a married man might go because he knows he can find a prostitute there. They may have known the prostitutes were men in women's clothing. Or they might not. It's quite possible they might never have known."

ELEVEN

Drug-Resistant Staphylococcus

March–June 2003,
Los Angeles

D<small>R. NOLAN LEE LOOKED DOWN</small> at the sheet that had just emerged from his desktop printer. It was late in a midweek workday in the first half of June. Outside Nolan's window, the dense gray cloud of Southern California's "June gloom" had turned glowing white as the sun moved behind it. On the elevated highway that passes the Los Angeles County Department of Health Services, late-afternoon traffic was clotting into the beginning of rush hour.

The list on the sheet Nolan was staring at represented the first pass through a computer program of a set of data he had gathered from local men. The men came from across Los Angeles, but they had several things in common. They were mostly gay. They were mostly HIV-positive. They were patients at several large medical practices in Hollywood. And for months, they had been turning up with stubborn skin infections that resisted treatment, ate away at tissue, and infected their blood and bones.

There was no mystery about the pathogen causing the problem. Lab tests had identified it as methicillin-resistant *Staphylococcus aureus,* a bug that had lurked in hospitals since the 1970s and had escaped in the 1990s into the wider community. The puzzle was why it was infecting these men in particular. Resistant staph aureus has a preference for tightly knit groups: Researchers had found it in dialysis patients, high school athletes, and extended families of immigrants. But the Los Angeles health authorities could find no reason why, this time, resistant staph had chosen to infect men who have sex with men.

The results on Nolan's list suggested a possible answer. Men in long-term relationships were less likely to be infected; men with multiple partners were more likely to have picked up the bug. The drug-resistant staph, usually passed by skin-to-skin contact or by surviving for awhile on an environmental surface, was behaving like a sexually transmitted disease.

The findings explained the problem. They also suggested the complex problems that lay ahead. Just as in the early days of AIDS twenty-two years before, a relatively straightforward public health investigation was about to collide with ideals of sexual freedom and the negotiations of local politics.

Lee picked up the list. "I think I'd better tell my supervisor," he said.

———

Nolan, a thirty-two-year-old family physician, had started thinking about the Epidemic Intelligence Service in high school, after reading a 1991 *National Geographic* article about epidemiologists. On the magazine's cover, a scientist peered out through the visor of the moon-suit protective gear used in the CDC's hot labs.

"I always remembered the space suits," Nolan said. "It was absolutely captivating to me."

Nolan was a Southern California native. His father, an engineer, had emigrated from China. His mother was an accountant and his younger brother a wildlife biologist. As an undergraduate at Berkeley, he had wavered between science and literature and ended up an English-biology double major.

"I was always going back and forth between science and writing," he said. "I wanted to be scientifically rigorous, and also communicate scientific findings in a way that would affect policy, and I couldn't find too many ways to do that. I thought about doing environmental science, so, one summer, I went to Costa Rica. I was sitting in the jungle, doing a survey of tree falls—that's where a falling tree creates a hole in the forest canopy, letting in light and increasing the biodiversity—and I thought: 'I really want something with more people in it.' So I applied to medical school."

Nolan retained his affection for literature; in Los Angeles, he signed the monthly memos he was required to write for Atlanta, describing what he was doing, with quotations from poems. (In April 2003, in the chaos of the SARS epidemic, he chose an excerpt from Stanley Kunitz's "Night Letter": "Cities shall suffer siege and some shall fall, / But man's not taken.") But he followed the traditional steps of medical education, going to medical school at Hahnemann University in Philadelphia and interning at San Francisco General Hospital. In San Francisco, he fell in love with a dermatologist headed for a residency at University of Illinois in Chicago. He finished his own residency, followed her north, and spent a year getting a public health degree and working in an urban family-practice clinic. They married in June 2002. The next month, he moved to Atlanta to start his EIS training, knowing he would be there for only four weeks.

The anthrax attacks of 2001 underlined how badly the states needed public health workers: Once the link between illnesses and contaminated letters was established, health departments were overwhelmed by calls from frightened citizens and reports of ominous letters that had to be analyzed even though they looked like hoaxes—and in almost every case turned out to be loaded with sugar, baby powder, or nothing at all. After the crisis was over, Secretary of Health and Human Services Tommy Thompson pledged to put an EIS officer in every state that wanted one. In a supplemental appropriation in spring 2002, Congress pumped enough additional money into the CDC's budget to create EIS positions in thirty-nine states, the largest number of assignments outside Atlanta ever offered to corps members.

Among them was a job working for Paul Simon, a former pediatrician, in a unit of the Los Angeles County health department that kept track of chronic diseases and toxic exposures. Nolan took the job as soon as it was offered. It let him live with his parents in Orange County while he waited for his wife to finish residency and join him. More important, it put him on the front line of public health. When something unusual happens, local health departments are the first to hear.

"When Atlanta gets a call from a state or local health department saying, 'We need help,' several people have already thought about it: Is this an outbreak? How big is it? What are the first steps we take?" said Elizabeth Bancroft, who was an EIS officer in Los Angeles three years before Nolan and stayed to work for the county when her term was up.

Bancroft had intended to be a surgeon until an accident rerouted her life. Halfway through residency, with a master's in epidemiology already completed, she won a prestigious scholarship to study in Asia for a year, and fell off a cliff on a hike several weeks after she arrived. She broke her back. She was medevac'd back to the United States, but after eighteen months of rehab could not regain the use of her legs. Specializing in surgery was impractical for a wheelchair user; she switched to preventive medicine, finished residency, and arrived in Los Angeles in the summer of 1999.

"I loved being the one who had to do all that initial thinking," she said. I got to pick up the phone and hear someone say, 'We think we have a situation here'"

In Los Angeles, Nolan was surrounded by people who had arranged their careers so that they would be the ones to pick up the phone. Simon, his boss, had been the only EIS officer in Colorado from 1990 to 1992; he had solved an outbreak of children's abscesses that turned out to be caused by accidental contamination in the alcohol used for sterilizing their skin before vaccinations. Laurene Mascola, Simon's counterpart—she headed Los Angeles' infectious-disease unit—had been one of the CDC's first AIDS investigators.

Nolan had come to California at a critical time. The state government was in crisis: Governor Gray Davis was facing a recall election and the budget was $8 billion in the red. The Department of Health Services, Nolan's new home, had announced plans to close a well-known hospital and had just laid off 100 employees. Urgent fliers from the employee unions advertising strategy sessions were taped to the elevator walls. An additional worker—especially one paid by the CDC—was just what the group needed. They threw assignments at him: a set of skin infections among a college football team; a survey of how overweight Los Angeles school kids were; a mysterious cluster of cases of sudden double vision, caused by unexplained palsies of the sixth cranial nerve.

The panic over the budget sharpened the always-fractious politics that swirl around public health issues. Behind the scrim of Southern California image, Los Angeles had the health problems of any urban area: obesity, cancer, smoking, heart disease, and a homicide rate twice as high as New York City's. But local health awareness and long-standing liberal tradition—and entertainment industry money—combined to layer an extra set of concerns on top of the traditional ones. The health department had recently failed to persuade studios to deglamorize smoking in movies. And when Nolan arrived in Los Angeles, environmental investigator and movie heroine Erin Brockovich and her associates had just filed suit over oil wells located next to Beverly Hills High School, contending that exposure to toxic emissions had caused cancers in several generations of students.

It was in that atmosphere—contentious, politicized, cautious about money—that Nolan picked up on the puzzling increase in skin infections in gay men.

"It was very casual, how it happened," he said. "An infectious-disease clinic had seen an increase in these infections, and they mentioned it to someone in our department, and we thought we should have a look. They had no idea what they had. They just knew they had a lot of it."

———

The pathogen behind the skin infections, methicillin-resistant *Staphylococcus aureus,* or MRSA, was a troublesome one. Staph aureus, a spherical bacterium that under a microscope bunches together like clusters of grapes, is everywhere in the environment. About one-third of the population carries it around on their skin or in their nostrils without ever being made sick by it, but it is a common cause of rapid-onset, violent food poisoning. When it invades the body, passing through the barriers posed by the surface of the skin and the lining of the gut and entering the bloodstream, staph causes much more serious illness: pneumonia, septicemia, and heart and bone infections. It is the most common cause of skin infections in the United States, and a persistent problem for hospitals and nursing homes because the sites where intravenous lines pierce the skin are particularly vulnerable to invasion by bacteria. More than 400,000 patients develop staph infections each year, usually after being infected in the hospital by health care workers who unknowingly carry the germ on their skin.

The bug was first kept in check by penicillin, which entered wide use in the United States after World War II. Within a decade of its introduction, though, some strains of the bacteria evolved defenses against the drug. Newer pharmaceuticals were developed. One was methicillin, from a group of synthetic cousins of penicillin called beta-lactams after a detail of their chemical structure.

"Methicillin was created in the early 1960s specifically in response to the rapid development of penicillin-resistant staph aureus," said Dr. Scott Fridkin, a CDC epidemiologist and ex-EIS officer who tracks the spread of MRSA in the United States. "Staph had been causing outbreaks in hospitals, and penicillin was used to treat them. So methicillin became the drug of choice against staph."

As soon as methicillin began to be used, staph bacteria began evolving defenses against it. The first U.S. case with some resistance to methicillin was diagnosed in 1968. Researchers soon discovered that the genetic change producing the resistance protected staph against more than just methicillin: It blocked the action of the entire class of beta-lactam drugs. Methicillin-resistant staph had evolved protection against not only the original wonder drug penicillin, but all its chemical cousins as well: cephalosporin, amoxicillin, cephalexin, nafcillin, and oxacillin. In the huge armamentarium of pharmaceuticals, only a few drugs remained that could have an impact on staph, and the bacteria were evolving resistance faster than drug companies could produce new compounds to combat it.

Over three decades, the newly strengthened bacteria popped up unpredictably worldwide, appearing in patients in Denmark, Belgium, Ireland, the Netherlands, and Australia as well as the United States. By 1997, half of all the staph infections that were acquired in intensive care units in U.S. hospitals were methicillin-resistant. Still, its influence seemed confined to health care institutions. Most of the time, it attacked adults and the elderly in intensive care units, nursing homes, and rehabilitation centers, places where patients were already very ill. Every so often, there was an anomalous case that had no clear link to a hospital. Each time, state health departments uncovered a connection to a health care worker, or a patient who was sick or had an implanted medical device. MRSA was not considered a risk for the average person.

Until August 1999. That month, the Minnesota Department of Health announced that in the past two years four children in the upper Midwest had died of overwhelming MRSA infection. The victims had little in common. Three lived in the countryside and one in a city; two were white, one was black, and one was Native American, and they ranged in age from twelve months to thirteen years. None of them had any connection to any of the others, or to anyone who had been hospitalized or worked in a health care institution. They represented the first recognized cases in a different MRSA epidemic: "community-acquired" infections that had no apparent connection to the health care world.

The bug causing the new outbreaks was different too. Molecular fingerprinting done at the CDC and elsewhere revealed that, though the bacteria infecting the four children were almost identical to each other, they were not the same as the MRSA strain common in U.S. hospitals. Researchers had already pinpointed the stretch of genetic material that conferred beta-lactam resistance; they had found three close variants of the genetic sequence, which they called "staphylococcal chromosomal cassette *mec*" for the key genes involved. The non-hospital cases of MRSA contained a fourth variant of the cassette, or string of genes; it was half the size of the other three.

The good news in that finding was that the bug was less drug-resistant than the hospital strain, possibly because the resistance sequence in the new MRSA strain was shorter. By the time of the children's deaths, 50 percent of MRSA infections in U.S. hospitals had evolved additional resistance mechanisms and could be treated reliably with only one drug, vancomycin. The community strain, it turned out, was vulnerable to a number of drugs, just not to beta-lactams.

But all four children had initially been given the beta-lactam cephalosporin when they were first hospitalized, because it was the first drug on the list for treating childhood infections suspected to be caused by staph. If the victims' doctors had known that MRSA existed outside hospitals, the CDC suggested in an analysis, they would have chosen appropriate drugs more rapidly, and the children might not have died.

The review of the cases, published in the CDC's weekly bulletin, sounded an ominous note. "The rural/urban and racial diversity among these cases suggest that MRSA colonization may be widespread," the authors warned. "The extent of community-acquired MRSA infection in the United States is unknown."

The bacteria themselves provided a partial answer. In the next three years, health authorities uncovered community-acquired MRSA among children in Chicago and Nashville, military personnel in Hawaii, Inuit steam-bath users in Alaska, Samoan immigrants in California, prison inmates in Mississippi, and high school athletes in Texas. They all shared the same symptoms: unexplained abscesses, boils, and suppurating skin rashes that arose quickly and were slow to heal.

Health authorities could find no links among the outbreaks. Community-acquired MRSA, it seemed, was arising in multiple places at the same time through the random roulette of genetic mutation. Researchers feared, though, that an additional factor might be at work. That was the bad news implicit in the finding that the new bug's resistance code was so much shorter: The cassette's smaller size might make it more mobile, allowing the resistance sequence to spread widely among strains of staph as they replicated. Researchers began to be concerned that the pace at which methicillin resistance was spreading would accelerate. They feared the resistant bug would become even more common and, as in the case of the Midwestern children, go unrecognized until potentially too late.

Then, in the summer of 2002, the Los Angeles County Jail reported that its inmates were complaining of spider bites.

The hulking gray building that squats south of Dodger Stadium has one of the largest jail populations in the country: 165,000 inmates move through it every year, with most of them staying for less than two months. Since September 2001, men and women incarcerated there had been complaining of small, sore, pimple-like eruptions that appeared without warning and rapidly got worse. As the complaints mounted, the jail authorities reacted. Inmates with bites were given antibiotics. Jail health workers took samples from the skin infections and cultured them to find out the infections' cause. An exterminator was hired to wipe out the spider infestation. The Los Angeles County entomologist was called in to consult.

The spiders, it turned out, were a non-biting variety. The inmates' wounds had taken so long to heal because their infections were immune to the antibiotics used to treat them. The jail had become the unwitting host for the largest single MRSA outbreak yet seen in the United States.

By the time the outbreak was discovered in June 2002, hundreds of inmates had picked up the infection. Some recovered quickly once proper antibiotics were given. Others became seriously ill. Several were hospitalized with infections of the heart or bone marrow, and others had to have large areas of infected and dead tissue surgically removed.

The Los Angeles County Health Department moved in on the outbreak, telling the jail to treat every wound found on an inmate as though it were contaminated with staph. The jail began to check inmates daily for infections, made sure they showered daily, disinfected the cells, clothing, and bedding of anyone diagnosed with MRSA, and tried to dissuade them from lancing boils and abscesses themselves, a maneuver that could spread the stubborn bacteria to other inmates and to the entire environment. Still the outbreak persisted. It would rack up almost 100 cases a month for more than a year.

"MRSA is a disease of skin-to-skin contact and poor hygiene," said Bancroft, who led the investigation. "A jail is the most perfect possible environment for spreading it. You have people in crowded living conditions. By California law, they only have to be offered showers three times a week, and they can refuse. They only get new underpants twice a week, and a new jumpsuit once a week. And we have people coming in and out, from all around the county. So we're constantly reseeding the population with MRSA."

The health department feared that MRSA would begin to show up elsewhere in Los Angeles. They were right. Several sheriffs' deputies were diagnosed with the bacteria; then a deputy's child became infected. MRSA spread to underage inmates in the county juvenile hall. Then the infection reached outside law enforcement. In one week, two members of a college football team were hospitalized with resistant staph infections. Looking back, Bancroft realized that four babies born earlier in the year had been victims as well. The investigator had thought the babies, all patients in a neonatal intensive care unit, had been infected inside the hospital. When she looked closer, sending off for the infants' test results in the hospital's records, she realized the babies had left the hospital healthy. They had been infected once they left the nursery; from five to thirteen days later, they returned with severe skin infections that required intravenous antibiotics to clean them up.

Once again, investigators found no links between the outbreaks, though they could not say for certain that no link existed.

"We don't have the personnel to find out," Bancroft said. "If we interviewed all one thousand people in the jail who had this, we might find one of them is a household member of someone who worked in the newborn nursery, or something like that. But I'm not sure we're actually going to be able to find perfect person-to-person links. There are too many variables. MRSA runs the gamut from people who are colonized with the bacteria but never develop symptoms, all the way up to infections of the heart and brain."

In the vocabulary of public health, MRSA is not a "reportable disease." Physicians are under no obligation to look for the bacterium or to tell health authorities when they have found it in a patient. So the Los Angeles health department had no reliable data that could tell them how widely MRSA had spread in their community, and no gauge for whether the situation was worse than at any time before. In the fall of 2002, though, they knew that whenever they looked for MRSA, they seemed to find it.

It showed up as well in some places they had not yet thought to look. In November 2002, four months after Nolan arrived in Los Angeles, doctors in two large infectious-disease practices contacted the health department. Among their clients, many of them gay men who were HIV-positive but taking multidrug regimens that kept their health stable, the physicians had started to see a rash of serious skin infections. They were accustomed to dealing with unpredictable problems, since HIV's undermining of the immune system leaves infected people vulnerable to microbes that a healthy person could fight off. But the lesions the physicians were seeing in their patients were unusual. They began as small spots resembling insect bites, but expanded rapidly into ugly boils and abscesses that ate away at tissue and had sent some men to the hospital for intensive treatment.

One of the first to sound the alarm was Peter Ruane of Tower Infectious Disease Associates, a physician-researcher who specializes in treating HIV-positive men.

"People started showing up with really aggressive soft-tissue infections—on the chest wall, in the armpit, in the groin, on the buttocks," he said. "They were very destructive. Really, some of them would take your breath away."

The infections were fast-moving: One patient complained that he had scratched himself one day and the next found an abscess the size of a quarter. And they spread rapidly. Another was diagnosed with an abscess on the right kneecap and then hospitalized when the infection spread from calf to thigh. He was treated with a combination of intravenous and oral antibiotics. Ten days after the course of drugs ended, he was back in the hospital, with painful, swollen sores on his abdomen, down both legs and inside his nose.

Ruane's wife, Margie Morgan, was a microbiologist in the pathology department of Cedars-Sinai Medical Center in Los Angeles. She ran analyses of the bug isolated from the men's infections. It was MRSA. Molecular fingerprinting proved it was essentially the same strain of MRSA as in the jail outbreak and the neonatal intensive care outbreak, and in almost every community outbreak of MRSA in the country over the past four years.

Troublingly, though, it was not exactly the same. Chromosomally, this organism was more virulent: It produced a potent additional toxin that created more cellular damage. The evidence from the patients confirmed the lab's findings: The staph circulating in Los Angeles seemed unusually aggressive. It didn't need to find a scrape or wound in order to establish an infection. Boils and abscesses were rising where there had been only intact, healthy skin.

———

Ruane and the other physicians who found the staph in their patients volunteered to help the health department figure out where it was coming from. With their patients' consent, the doctors enrolled them in a study written by Nolan. For every man with a staph infection, the researchers picked another participant who was not infected, but was otherwise as much like the first man as possible.

The research team knew from other outbreaks that staph passes between people by contact with skin, or with an environmental surface. They knew that in newly infected people, the first lesions would show up close to where the bacteria made contact with the skin. And they knew that in the clinics' patients, staph eruptions were showing up in a distinctive pattern: primarily on the abdomen and buttocks, and near the genitals and anus. In one of Ruane's patients, the infection began on his scrotum. He ended up in intensive care.

The evidence suggested two hypotheses: The men were picking up the bacteria either from a surface they encountered while they were naked—a gym towel, for instance, or a steam-bath bench—or from skin-to-skin contact while they had sex. To figure out which, the health department needed more data. To get it, Nolan needed to know what questions to ask.

So on a Saturday evening in the spring, Nolan found himself in one of the front rooms of a bath house in West Hollywood, clutching a towel in one hand and waiting for a state health department colleague who had promised to show him around. Nolan—heterosexual, married, and affectionately described by classmates as "innocent"—had never been in a gay bath house before.

His colleague made that clear the moment they met. He looked the fully dressed Nolan up and down and grinned. "Let's go to the locker room," he said. "You're supposed to leave your clothes there, and wear only the towel."

The bath house the two had chosen had a door at the back, shielded from the street, that opened into a cashier's cubicle sheathed in bulletproof glass. Beyond the lockers were a series of mirrored, windowless rooms that led to a steam room, a pool, and a patio with a hot tub. Off to the sides were cubicles that could be rented for several hours; each one held a cot, and a door that latched from the inside. Men looking for a sexual encounter would sit or lie in the cubicle, waiting for an interested patron to walk by and look in.

Nolan wandered through the maze, taking mental notes, tightening the towel he had wrapped around his waist and trying not to feel voyeuristic, or naïve. "It was important to understand the environment," he said. "I couldn't see asking someone questions without knowing what I'm talking about."

Nolan made visits to several clubs. The visits led to a series of questions that he asked the men who agreed to be interviewed: Had they shared a towel with someone else? Had they used a sauna or a hot tub? Did they share sex toys or lubricant? Did they have sex through a "glory hole," an opening cut into a panel that masked the identity of the man on the other side? Were they drug users? Had they ever been urinated on?

When he had gathered answers from almost 120 men, Nolan ran his first preliminary analysis. The program quickly drew associations between the bits of data. Men were more likely to be infected if they hooked up with sex partners over the Internet; if they participated in group sex; if they used street drugs, especially inhibition-reducing speed and orgasm-enhancing nitrite inhalants. Men in long-term relationships were less likely to have been infected. The group at highest risk were those who had been to a bath house or a sex club in the past three months.

The findings made it clear that there was a tie between sexual activity and the risk of acquiring MRSA. But they had not answered a vital question: Was sex itself causing the infections? Or was it the surroundings that the sex was taking place in?

If the staph was being passed solely by skin-to-skin contact—between adults, in private—there was little the health department could do. They could post warnings in clubs and bath houses, trying to educate the people who might be at risk. But controlling diseases associated with sex is one of the most challenging tasks in public health, and carries a low likelihood of success. While Nolan was doing his study, HIV cases were climbing in the United States despite more than two decades of aggressive public education efforts aimed at limiting the spread of AIDS. Nor was HIV the only disappointment: Despite more than a century of public health efforts, syphilis had never been fully controlled.

But if the reservoir of infection was in the clubs themselves—in badly washed towels, perhaps, or vinyl benches that had not been cleaned—the authorities might have some leverage. Exercising it was risky, though: In a sophisticated city with a large gay population, appearing to restrict opportunities for sexual activity would win the health department no friends.

Nolan was too young to remember the political firestorm triggered twenty years earlier by San Francisco politicians who closed down that city's bathhouses to slow down the spread of AIDS. Melanie Taylor, a doctor in Los Angeles' STD unit, recounted the history to him. "The clubs are icons of sexual freedom," she said. "They're seen as one of the few places where gay men can't be touched by societal prejudice. They are quite resistant to regulation."

Taylor had reason to be concerned. Relationships between the STD unit and the commercial sex venues in Los Angeles had been touchy for a decade. In 1992, politicians worried by enthusiasm for barebacking, unprotected anal sex, had obtained a court injunction forcing clubs and bath houses to post rules of conduct and offer clients free condoms and lubricant. Under pressure from the city and from within the gay community, the clubs had complied. In recent years, some of them had allowed nonprofit groups to conduct STD testing and counseling inside.

Nevertheless, when Los Angeles public health investigators tried to track down the contacts of new syphilis cases, they found that one-third of them were still acquiring the disease at a bath house or a sex club. "The encounters are anonymous, unprotected, and multiple," Taylor said. "We have no way of contacting them. Our traditional public health control measures break down."

The day after Nolan drew his preliminary analysis, he and Simon huddled with Taylor, Bancroft, and Jorge Montoya, an investigator who worked closely with the clubs. Nolan and Simon wanted to find a way to check the bath house environments for staph, by swabbing benches and surfaces and analyzing the results for bacteria. The others, concerned by possible political fallout, wanted to debate the idea.

"Do we have the legal standing to come in unannounced and take cultures that could implicate them in an outbreak, when all our reports are public record?" Bancroft asked.

"I think we have the authority," Simon said. "The question is— given the relationships we've built up, given the sensitivity—whether we want to."

Bancroft frowned. "But if we find it in the environment, that doesn't mean it's causal," she pointed out. "We know there are multiple ways to catch this disease. It's not like syphilis, where there is only one way to acquire it."

Sampling the clubs was an attractive idea: If the cultures came up positive, the group could say they had tracked the stubborn bacteria to at least one of its hiding places. But it posed a practical problem: Should they call the clubs and ask their permission to conduct testing there? Or would Nolan have to arrive without warning, storming the cashier's desk with an armful of sample tubes and swabs?

"If you tell them, they will douse the place with bleach," Taylor warned. "The clubs are very competitive with each other, and they have had a lot of bad press. This is an issue of their brand."

Sampling raised an issue of fairness as well. If the researchers found the bacteria in a club, and disclosed its presence, the public would consider the club responsible. But the investigators had neither the time nor the personnel to conduct an exhaustive study. What if they missed a cluster of bacteria, and declared a place clean when it was actually colonized with staph? What if a club bench had been contaminated by an already-infected patron, and not the other way around?

"I was in favor of environmental testing," Bancroft admitted. "But if we find the staph there, what do we do with that?"

"When we haven't looked at gyms," Simon agreed.

"When we know it's been in a football team," Bancroft added. "There are kids who have this all across this city, and I know they're not getting it from a commercial sex venue. If you find it in a club, I don't think it will tell us anything except that it's there."

"But it helps target our efforts," Nolan pointed out.

"Does it?" she asked. "We still don't know, if it's found in the environment, that that is how people are acquiring it."

Taylor and Montoya, anxious not to disturb the fragile accord with the clubs unless really necessary, studied Nolan's analysis again.

"I think the link is sexual behavior," Taylor said. "I thought so from the beginning, but now I'm convinced. These data look like syphilis data to me."

"It's there in the environment," Bancroft agreed. "But that's not why they're getting it. They're getting it because they're high on drugs and doing multiple partners. It's the venue that allows them access to the drugs and multiple partners, but the issue isn't the venue itself."

———

In the end, the group decided against environmental testing, rejecting both consulting with the club owners and conducting commando-style raids. Instead, they voted for writing environmental guidelines that described the dangers of MRSA, explained how it could lurk in the environment, and prescribed thorough methods for keeping towels, benches, and equipment clean. The guidelines would be sent to all the sex clubs, and also to fitness gyms, athletic facilities, and anywhere else there might be a link to the disease.

Better methods of cleaning would not end the outbreak, the group agreed, though it might mitigate it. But MRSA had spread too far in Los Angeles to be reined in by any single initiative. Gay men were one of the groups hit hard by the disease, but not the only one. After L.A. County made pediatric MRSA reportable, Bancroft began getting calls every week about children hospitalized with the infection. In the week Nolan ran his data, the health service at University of California-Los Angeles admitted two college students who had picked up the bacteria, though no one knew where.

"This is not like a foodborne outbreak, where you find the source of the contamination and you shut the outbreak down," Nolan conceded. "It's an emerging disease that is finding its niche in the community."

"The bottom line," Bancroft said, "is that we have to assume it's everywhere."

Nolan was disappointed; like any physician, he was biased in favor of acting rather than waiting. But he understood the underlying point: The data were not yet solid enough to trump the attendant political difficulties. To move on the sex clubs and bath houses would have been satisfying, but it would not—from what they knew now—have been fair. And until he knew more, he could not predict with any certainty how much difference putting pressure on the clubs might make. He needed more data. He made plans to go back to Ruane and the other physicians to enroll more of their patients in his study, and to refine the analytical methods he used. With every additional person he could persuade to complete the study questionnaire, he would gain a small degree of statistical precision.

Simon, his supervisor, listened sympathetically to the plan.

"One of the things every EIS officer experiences—and Nolan had to learn this too—is that a field investigation is never as clean as a research study," Simon said. "It's messy. It's not well-controlled. It can be frustrating."

TWELVE

Terrorism

2001, New York City
and Washington, D.C.

WHEN THEY HAD A CHANCE TO LOOK BACK, everyone remembered that
it had been a beautiful day. The sky was a pure blue arch, unmarred
by cloud. It was warm—in Atlanta, early September is an extension of
summer—but there was a cool breeze freshening. The trees were all
green; only a few of the dogwoods showed a tinge of red along the
edges of their leaves. All the way up the Eastern Seaboard, the
weather was perfect.

At the CDC, Doug Hamilton was late for Tuesday morning seminar, the mandatory grand rounds for EIS members. The seminar was
always held in Auditorium B on the streetfront side of the campus. It
was the CDC's fanciest conference room, the place where dignitaries
were welcomed and new EIS classes took their summer training. It
had rows of movable chairs, blond wood walls and a ceiling made of
rippling, curved acoustical panels that looked like an abstract sculp-
ture. Its central feature was a huge projection screen that stretched

across the back of the stage. When EIS members made presentations about their investigations, audiovisual technicians in a darkened-glass booth built into the room's left wall threw their PowerPoint slides on the screen. When they took questions about their research, the technicians patched in a videoconference link to other CDC locations, and projected the questioners' images on the screen instead.

Tuesday morning seminar always begins at 9:00 a.m. Hamilton arrived about three minutes afterward. As he pulled open the double doors at the back of the auditorium, his boss, Dr. Stephen Thacker, caught up with him and held him back.

"A plane has hit the World Trade Center," Thacker said. "Should we make an announcement?"

Hamilton envisioned a small touring plane losing its bearings in the visual flight corridor down the center of the Hudson and hitting the side of the city's tallest buildings. He shook his head. "There's nothing we can do," he said. "Let's go on with the seminar."

Hamilton slid into a seat in the back row. Ten minutes later, one of the video technicians tapped him on the shoulder from behind. "Another plane just hit the World Trade Center," the man whispered.

Disbelieving, Hamilton got up and followed him into the control room. On their desk screens, the technicians had turned off the PowerPoint feed and switched to CNN. The channel was running the same loop of tape, over and over: The first jet, slamming into Tower One of the World Trade Center; the flash of its disintegration; the plume of smoke boiling slowly across the clear blue sky. Underneath the image, the news crawl ticked by: Passenger plane hits World Trade Center, 8:46 a.m.; second plane crashes, 9:02 a.m.

Hamilton watched the loop a dozen times, trying to absorb what he was seeing. Shaken and dazed, he walked back to his seat. Thacker was across the auditorium, next to retired CDC director David Sencer; they always sat in the same spot, halfway up the aisle on the right-hand side. Next to Hamilton's empty seat, though, Dr. Denise Koo had settled into the back row. She was in the same division and between Hamilton and Thacker on the organizational chart.

"You're not going to believe what's happening," he said to her.

The two were deep into a whispered conversation when the technician nudged Hamilton again. It was not long after 9:40 a.m. He didn't bother to lower his voice this time.

"A plane has hit the Pentagon," he said.

The seminar stopped. The speaker sat down. The technicians threw CNN on the huge video screen. The staff in the auditorium, and the ones on the other end of the video links, watched in silence. A few of them left to make family phone calls. A few cried.

Tower Two of the World Trade Center collapsed at 9:59 a.m. Tower One fell thirty minutes later.

By the time the second tower collapsed, Hamilton was back in his fifth-floor office two buildings away, gathering emails and phone numbers of members of the corps. What was unfolding was a national emergency. The EIS existed to serve in such emergencies. He was sure the group would be summoned to action—though, watching the endlessly replaying tape of the collapsing towers, he was not sure what they could do.

The chime of a high-priority email cut across the mutter of the television. A plane without a flight plan had been detected heading toward Atlanta. The CDC was being evacuated.

———

Marci Layton had come to work early that morning. She was giving three speaches in Canada the next day, and she wanted to get her slides in order. The workload in the New York City Department of Health was so intense that she knew she would have no spare time once the daily round of calls and meetings started.

Layton was one of the department's assistant commissioners and the chief of its bureau of communicable diseases. She had just passed forty, a slender, energetic woman with curly, center-parted light brown hair and huge blue eyes. She was a graduate of Duke Medical School who had done residency in Syracuse and an infectious disease fellowship at Yale. In between academic stints, she had volunteered in clinics in Nepal, Thailand, and Alaska.

She had worked in the ten-story white marble pile with the octagonal brass door handles embossed "City of New York" for nine years, since arriving in the summer of 1992 as an EIS officer. By chance, her predecessor in her Yale fellowship turned out to have gone into EIS two years before her. He had taken the New York posting and prevailed on her to take it too: In New York City, he said, every disease she had seen in the Third World would show up on her doorstep.

The New York health department was such a good fit that, when her EIS stint ended in 1994, Layton agreed to stay. Her predecessor's prediction proved correct: New York had almost one hundred disease emergencies a year, ranging from foodborne diseases to an outbreak of malaria to a stubborn tuberculosis epidemic. There were other emergencies also. In February 1993, terrorists set off bombs in a parking lot beneath the World Trade Center ten blocks from the health department, killing six and injuring more than a thousand. And in August 1999, dozens of New York residents sickened abruptly with encephalitis in what turned out to be the first outbreak of West Nile virus in the Americas.

The health department building lies in lower Manhattan, south of Chinatown and north of Wall Street. It is a part of the city that is seldom quiet. Trucks rumble by day and night, heading for the ramps of the Manhattan and Brooklyn bridges. A subway line runs directly underneath the building. Planes on approach to LaGuardia and Kennedy pass constantly overhead. Still, the boom that shook Layton's office about an hour after her arrival was disorientingly loud. It sounded, she thought, as though a plane had crashed.

Shortly afterward, her phone rang. It was her parents in Baltimore; they wanted her to know her sister had had a baby overnight, and they wanted to be sure she was okay.

Their concern cut through her confusion. She walked to the other side of the building, to windows that faced southwest. She saw the gaping holes in the sides of the towers and the fires bellying out of them. Bodies were beginning to fall from the floors above.

The next time she had a moment to look out the window, it was 2:00 a.m.

In the panic that followed the attacks, it was hard to get a grip on what was happening. TV reception went out when the buildings fell.

Electrical power was patchy, and so was cell phone reception. The wired phones died at 2:00 p.m. The health department assumed the towers' collapse would bring thousands of people streaming into emergency rooms. They sent staff out to walk to the closest hospitals, to log the injuries and to see what extra staff and supplies the institutions needed. The answer was very little. Over two days, four ERs and a burn center saw only 1,688 patients. Most of them arrived within eight hours of the attacks; three-fourths of them were able to walk into the emergency room and to walk away again afterward. Calls to all the other hospitals in the city confirmed the picture that was emerging. The injured were mostly not survivors from the towers; they were passers-by, or first responders who had rushed downtown. Thousands of people had made it out of the buildings, but they had all worked below the crash sites.

The vast majority trapped above, on seventeen floors of Tower One and thirty-two floors of Tower Two, had died.

Since there was no wave of trauma victims that would overwhelm city hospitals, the health department turned to the next set of problems: air quality, water safety, getting care to the homebound elderly and disabled. Restaurant customers and staff in the financial district had fled, leaving food on the tables; it was a buffet for rats and insects emboldened by the lack of people in the stores and streets. And there was a further lurking concern. Since the Trade Center bombing in 1993, law enforcement, the health department, and the city's emergency management office had war-gamed possible terrorist attacks. They had predicted that a conventional assault would be followed by a second, unconventional one, something insidious, something that would be masked by the chaos and disruption. Bioterrorism was their best guess.

At 2:00 a.m. on September 12, Layton and her colleagues met in her office to figure out how to detect a bioterrorist attack before it spawned an epidemic. They had to assume it would come with a whimper, not a bang—not a hundred cases of disease in a single place, but a few patients in one emergency room and a single one in another, or in a doctor's office, or a street corner clinic. Those were places that had no connection to each other and would not recognize they were part of a brewing outbreak until after the cases they had missed had infected many other.. Layton needed a way to identify those potential patients, no matter where they were in the city, as soon as they sought help.

New York already had a system that detected public health anomalies, a computer program that analyzed ambulance transport records to spot emerging trends. But the availability of ambulances had been disrupted by the chaos in the city. Patients arriving at emergency rooms were getting there on their own.

The alternative was actually putting health department representatives into emergency rooms to gather data from doctors as patients were being evaluated. It had been tried before, at the Winter Olympics and national political conventions; it seemed to work, though there had never been any bioterrorist attacks to test it. But it was cumbersome, and hugely labor intensive. The health department had nowhere near enough personnel to make it work.

Layton called the CDC in Atlanta, and asked it to send whatever EIS officers as it could spare. Then she evacuated her own office. The smoke and debris and the lack of phones and power had made it uninhabitable; the department was moving en masse to its own laboratory building at Twenty-sixth Street, thirty blocks uptown.

———

Scott Harper had been in the Tuesday seminar when the images of the Trade Center flashed on the screen and the auditorium fell silent. He had watched for a while, until the magnitude of the attacks became clear. By the time the call came to empty the CDC buildings, he had gone home to be with his wife Stephanie and their two-year-old daughter. He also had started packing. He was a second-year EIS officer, and he expected to be mobilized.

Harper was an infectious-disease physician, born in San Antonio and trained in Dallas and San Francisco. He and Stephanie, an audiologist, had met in high school and been together since college. After his residency, they had gone abroad for three years, working in clinics in Cambodia, India, Togo, and South Africa, and then spending a year in London while Scott got a public health degree. Now he was thirty-six, but looked younger. He had a rounded face and brown hair that flopped over his forehead, and he wore chunky-knit sweaters that rolled back on themselves at the neck and cuffs.

When the CDC was evacuated, the senior leadership had relocated to an emergency operations center on the Chamblee campus. The property was larger, and more defensible if necessary, and unlike the Clifton Road headquarters was not surrounded by houses and university dorms. Hamilton had gone with them. The plane thought to be heading for Atlanta had turned out to be a false alarm, so the CDC's main campus reopened one day later. The ops center stayed in Chamblee, running around the clock in twelve-hour shifts.

Two EIS officers and four other CDC staff members had left for New York within hours of the attacks, hitching a ride on a cargo plane carrying a load of pharmaceuticals and medical supplies. Dozens more had volunteered to go next. On the evening of the 12th, Hamilton sent out an email asking who could leave for New York in the next twenty-four hours. When he opened his email the next morning, there were fifty responses in his inbox. Scott had sent one of them.

Layton did not need fifty, at least not at first. She had decided to focus on fifteen key hospitals in the five New York boroughs, places where someone seriously ill might seek care. She asked the CDC for about thirty officers, two per hospital, to work twelve-hour shifts. By the time the CDC got the EIS members to New York, the department would know exactly what questions they wanted asked in the emergency rooms.

The EIS needed to bring laptops, so patient data could be recorded on the spot and transferred easily to the health department. It was a simple-sounding requirement, but when the volunteers gathered in Auditorium B on Thursday evening to be briefed, it proved difficult to fulfill. The EIS's congressionally set budget had been flat-funded for several years in a row; for the same several years, there had been no money for new equipment. The laptops the corps members had been given had been passed on from earlier classes and were aging and balky. To make sure all the New York data would match, the laptops all had to contain the same version of one software program; one after another, though, the machines froze, crashed, and choked on the download. Watching the IT workers struggle, Hamilton realized that he had bigger technology problems. Most of the corps had personal cell phones, but they might be going into areas of the city where the cell networks were dead. A few of them had been given pagers by their offices, but none of them were two-way pagers. He had no time—and no money and no government-approved purchase order— to get them anything better. If the disease detectives ran into trouble while they were in the city, they would be on their own until they could find a working wired phone.

Getting them to New York proved to be the easy part. U.S. air travel had been grounded since the attacks. That took out not only commercial carriers, but the charters the CDC sometimes relied on. Calling around Atlanta, the agency found a last-minute alternative. At the Lockheed Martin Aeronautics Co. plant in Marietta, on the northwest corner of metro Atlanta, a C-130 belonging to the Royal Australian Air Force was undergoing software upgrades. The crew who had accompanied it were not bound by the restrictions on American flag carriers. They leapt at the chance to help.

The thirty volunteers left early the next morning. They assembled at the CDC to be bused to the Lockheed air strip. CDC director Jeffrey Koplan, on crutches from recent foot surgery, stood at the door to shake their hands as they went by. Once they were in the air, the Australian pilots came back to greet them. President George W. Bush was on his way to New York to visit the Trade Center site; aside from Air Force Once and its fighter escorts, the pilots said, they were the only plane in the air anywhere above America.

A few hours later, they were at LaGuardia. As they walked off the tarmac, Scott noticed that something felt wrong. It took him a minute to realize what the problem was. The usually bustling airport, normally one of the busiest in the country, was silent.

The problem with detecting bioterrorism was that it was likely to look, at first, like a number of other illnesses. The viruses and bacteria most feared by planners could cause fever, rashes, headaches, or diarrhea before they progressed enough to reveal themselves as smallpox, botulism, tularemia, or plague. The initial complaints were so non-specific that any single doctor might see them on any day. The challenge was separating the worrisome cases from the innocuous ones, uncovering the bioterror-related cases as they were emerging.

While the EIS was getting ready to leave Atlanta, Layton and her staff had drafted a questionnaire for them to use in the emergency rooms, a single page that asked about sets of symptoms including breathing difficulties, gut complaints, coughing and trouble breathing, headache and stiff neck, and rashes accompanied by fever. The health department workers met the volunteers at the airport, ferried them to the department's temporary quarters for a briefing, and then drove them out to the hospitals, stacks of pink questionnaires in hand.

The forms were designed to be filled out by nurses or doctors who saw ER patients, and then handed to the CDC volunteers to be recorded in a database. It did not go as planned. The ER personnel left the forms incomplete, or neglected them entirely. After a few disappointing days, the volunteers resorted to grabbing the patients' medical charts, paging through them for doctors' notes on vital signs and symptoms, and filling out the forms and the matching database entries themselves. Shifts lasted twelve hours; at the end of every shift, the EIS officers loaded whatever they had gathered onto a diskette, hitched a ride back to First Avenue and Twenty-sixth Street, and handed over the data to be processed before the next set came in. Then they hiked uptown, where the health department had put them up in a hotel.

It was difficult, being in the city. Mass transit was cut back, so there were few commuters and fewer pedestrians. There were police or National Guard at major intersections. As far north as Canal Street, streets were sealed off to vehicles. Light poles and bus shelters were papered over with the flyers that family members had posted in the first chaotic hours, flyers that everyone soon understood bore the faces of the dead. At the tip of the island, the Trade Center site smoked and steamed. When the wind blew north, it carried smoke with it, and a bitter tang like a radio burning.

Some of the corps members had volunteered to work at the site, to gauge the air quality and make sure rescue personnel were wearing protective gear. The rest tried to get there whenever they could, to help, to pay their respects, or simply to bear witness. For more than a week afterward, there were body parts visible in the rubble, and on most days, bodies of firefighters who had been trapped in the towers' collapse were brought out. On the way into his hotel one day, Scott stopped to allow a fireman's funeral to go past. The coffin had been loaded on a fire truck; a firefighter stood beside it, with one hand on the coffin and the other on his heart.

All over the city, it was quiet. It was quiet in the emergency rooms as well. In normal times, ERs are the doctors' offices of New York, full of people with all kinds of problems, from heart attacks to broken bones to flu.

"They weren't there," said Scott, who had been posted to Elmhurst Hospital Center in Queens. "The people with the general maladies stayed home. It was like the rest of the city, quiet; it took a few weeks for the traffic to pick up again."

It did pick up: Over four weeks, at fifteen hospitals, the EIS members took down details on 67,536 patients. Every few days, the computer programs examining the data sounded an alert: eight times for a higher than expected number of cases of rashes and fever, respiratory infection, and GI illness; sixteen times because there seemed to be too many cases in a single hospital; nine times because an unusual number of patients came from the same zip code. All were false alarms.

Layton began to be worried about the pace of the work. With the twelve-hour shifts and the cumbersome commutes, some corps members were getting only four hours of sleep a night. "We were burning them out," she said. "We decided to send them all home, and ask for more."

On September 26, Scott went back to Atlanta. The next day, twenty more CDC employees arrived in the city to spell their colleagues. Kelly Moore took over Scott's post at Elmhurst. Kelly was a first-year EIS officer, a pediatrician who had interrupted her residency to switch fields because she had become so enchanted with public health. She was from northern Alabama, a slight strawberry blonde who joked that Yankees expected her to have a Bible in one hand and a rifle in the other. Her parents raised beef cattle on a farm so close to Huntsville that they could see the rockets at the Space Center from their front gate.

Kelly had only been back in the country a week. On September 11, she had been in Cairo on her first EIS deployment, trying to uncover why half of the babies in a hospital's neonatal intensive care nursery were dying of overwhelming bacterial infections. She and a colleague, Marian Kainer, suspected the babies' IVs had been contaminated by nurses who did not wash their hands often enough. They found out about the attacks in an email message from a professor in New York who was sending them a recipe for hand-sanitizing gel: "I guess you heard about our disaster by now," it said.

They had not. They switched off the computer, turned on CNN, and sat on the bed and wept for hours. Then they tried to get home, only to find that international flights were not being allowed in U.S. airspace. They stayed, and kept working—solving the outbreak, but growing increasingly nervous about moving around Cairo—until the CDC found them a flight on September 20.

By the time Kelly took over from Scott, the New York health department had cut the shifts back to eight hours, though it had kept the requirement that each shift's worth of data had to be hand-carried to the statisticians. Kelly picked up where Scott had left off, dogging the steps of the emergency department doctors and nurses to make them fill out the pink sheets, and riffling through the patients' charts herself when they did not.

She did that for a week, and then everything changed. Like a magician pulling off a magic trick, bioterrorism struck exactly where they were not looking.

———

On September 30, a newspaper photo editor named Bob Stevens who lived in Lantana, Florida, abruptly came down with a fever and chills. Two days later, he grew so disoriented that his wife took him to the emergency department. Within a few hours, he had a seizure and lapsed into a coma. Doctors thought at first that he had meningitis. They gave him a diagnostic X-ray, which showed a peculiar widening of the mediastinum, a vertical space between the lungs that houses the heart, the major blood vessels and nerve trunks, and clusters of lymph nodes. When they tapped his spinal fluid and stained it to look for the organism that was making him sick, they found chains of distinctive, rod-shaped bacteria that gleamed purple with one of the stains they had used. Very few bacteria possessed that shape and responded in that manner to that particular stain. The lead candidate was *Bacillus anthracis,* the cause of anthrax disease.

Anthrax was a rare occurrence in humans in the United States. It was also one of the pathogens most likely to be used as a bioterrorism agent.

Dr. Larry Bush, the infectious-disease specialist whom the hospital summoned to consult on Stevens's case, called the Palm Beach County health department director. She had the samples rushed to Florida's state public health lab. They found the same bacteria. After a Florida FBI agent drove through the night to deliver a small sample of Stevens's cerebrospinal fluid, the CDC did as well. By then, it was early October 4, a Thursday. That afternoon, Health and Human Services Secretary Tommy Thompson stepped into the daily briefing of reporters at the White House, announced Stevens's illness, and suggested that the outdoors-loving Englishman had contracted the disease naturally, perhaps by drinking from a woodland stream in North Carolina, where he had been vacationing the week before he got sick. The case, along with Thompson's hypothesis, was the lead story on every evening newscast.

Kelly watched the news in the break room in the Elmhurst emergency department, along with several of the doctors. One of them looked over at her.

"Natural?" he asked. "I don't think so."

Clearly he was inviting comment from the CDC representative; only, she had no comment to give. "I don't know anything," she said. "This is the first I'm hearing about it."

The phone rang shortly afterward. It was Layton's office, with a new assignment: Forget about the pink sheets. Find out if any hospital patients in New York have the same symptoms that Stevens does.

The problem was not merely that Stevens's illness was rare. It was that it was extraordinarily rare. Anthrax usually infects cattle and goats. Because the bacteria form hard-shelled spores when exposed to air, anthrax can persist in the environment, such as the spot where a sick animal collapses, for a very long time. Anthrax bacteria occasionally cause illness in humans, usually in people who have had close contact with live animals, butchered ones, or skins or pelts. Most commonly, anthrax is a skin disease that causes a wide lesion with a coal-black crust ("anthracis" comes from the Greek word for coal). Up to one in five cases of cutaneous anthrax can be fatal. Less frequently, anthrax causes a gastrointestinal illness, which arises from eating meat contaminated with spores or bacteria; gastrointestinal anthrax is fatal about 50 percent of the time, but it occurs mostly in the developing world. Finally there was inhalational anthrax, the form of the disease Stevens had developed: a rapidly moving whole-body infection that originated in the lymph nodes linked to the lungs after bacteria were inhaled. Inhalational anthrax was fatal at least 85 percent of the time. Clinically, it followed a predictable pattern: one to four days of fatigue, fever, aches, and cough; a brief period of feeling better; then a crash, with sweating, dusky skin, and inability to breathe. Once the crash began, victims died within two days.

There had not been a case of inhalational anthrax in the United States since 1976, and only eighteen cases in the entire twentieth century. That made Stevens's case a medical mystery. But something else made his case an occasion for alarm and horror: Military planners had long speculated that, if anthrax were used as a biological weapon, it would be released in a way that would create cases of inhalational disease.

Kelly spent the night calling ERs and intensive care units around New York City, searching for patients with the same set of symptoms: rapid onset of fever, neurological disease, widened mediastinum on X-ray, rod-shaped bacteria that responded positively to Gram stain. By the next morning, she reported with relief that there were no known cases of inhalational anthrax in the five boroughs of New York.

That same day, Bob Stevens died. Simultaneously, though the CDC would not know it for several more days, Stevens' co-worker Ernesto Blanco was also hospitalized with the symptoms of inhalational anthrax. Blanco was seventy-three, a retiree who had gone back to work. He was a mail clerk at American Media Inc., the Boca Raton supermarket-tabloid publisher where Stevens was employed as well.

News of the Florida cases jolted New York just as the shock of the Trade Center attacks was beginning to leak away. On Monday, Columbus Day, the FBI called Layton to an emergency, a letter that contained an unidentified white powder. It was a busy day for emergencies. Several hours earlier, a physician had reported an unexplained case of fever and rash that he feared might be smallpox. The physician was wrong, though it took Layton several hours to be sure. She had barely returned to her temporary office when an FBI agent in an unmarked car arrived to pick her up. They roared uptown, blaring a siren. It took the rest of the day for Layton to be sure the letter was a hoax. The FBI took her back downtown, without sirens this time. It was dark by the time she arrived back at her office, and shortly afterward her cell phone rang. It was the FBI, again. They wanted Layton to call a thirty-six-year-old woman named Erin O'Connor, an assistant to NBC News anchor Tom Brokaw. O'Connor had heard the news from Florida. She had researched the disease over the weekend, and she thought she might have anthrax.

O'Connor was not seriously ill in the way that Stevens had been ill. Her symptoms were fever and a skin rash, which a doctor had already treated. But like Stevens, she worked in a large media organization and handled mail, and the coincidence made her anxious.

Skin samples were rushed to the New York City lab, and to the CDC. At 3:00 a.m. on October 12, several CDC scientists and its director, Koplan, eyed the samples through a microscope. The samples had been subjected to a test developed by CDC pathologists that would turn any anthrax bacteria bright red. O'Connor had been given antibiotics by the doctor treating her, but the drugs had not yet reached full effect. Through the eyepieces, the red signal showed clearly. O'Connor had cutaneous anthrax.

The health department announced her case later that morning. By the time Layton returned to her office at 7:00 p.m., after a long day of setting up the investigation at NBC and talking to its reporters and other media, she had dozens of phone messages and emails. Among them were news of three more anthrax cases, at CBS News, the *New York Post,* and ABC News, where the seven-month-old child of an assistant to news anchor Peter Jennings had become seriously ill after a ninety-minute visit to the building.

The anthrax situation could no longer be understood as a medical mystery limited to Florida. With news of the multiple New York cases, authorities had no choice but to construe the situation as an attack.

In midtown, Kelly had been packing to leave for Atlanta the next morning. At about midnight, a fax slid under her hotel room door.

"Your departure is cancelled," it read. "Please report to NBC News at 8 tomorrow morning."

———

The next morning, health department and CDC employees headed to all four media companies. At Rockefeller Center, the health department sealed off one floor of the NBC offices and triaged more than 1,200 employees into groups: the ones closest to where the sick woman worked, who needed to be checked for exposure and given antibiotics, and a much larger group who did not appear to qualify for protective drugs, but needed to be informed and reassured.

When Kelly arrived the next morning, informing became her job.

"They paired each of us with a crisis counselor, someone who had experience working with people in disasters," she said. "They handed us all the information the health department knew at that point about anthrax, and then they started to bring groups in, six or seven people at a time."

But—on that first day at least—the NBC employees had little interest in the crisis counseling. Emotional processing would come later; right now they wanted information, and Kelly had it. Over and over, she rehearsed the same points: Their co-worker had developed cutaneous anthrax, not the more dangerous inhalational kind. The CDC believed that, to develop a fatal case of inhalational anthrax, it was necessary to inhale thousands of bacterial spores. There was no evidence any of them had been exposed to a source of the spores. There was a test that could show whether there had been spores in the environment close to them, a "nasal swab"—shorthand for swabbing the inside of the nostrils, swishing the swab on a culture medium, and waiting to see if anything grew—but the test could not predict who would develop anthrax disease, and was imperfect even at indicating exposure. There was one solid protection against developing anthrax, taking up to sixty days of antibiotics; but the two main antibiotics were hard to tolerate and had a high rate of adverse reactions. Unless someone knew they had been exposed or had definite symptoms—fever, rashes, the beginnings of something that felt like flu—taking the drugs was not recommended.

Over three days, she repeated those messages to almost three hundred people. Some listened carefully to the detailed rundown of the differences among anthrax disease types and their fatality rates. Others were half out of their minds with anxiety over symptoms that might have been early-season colds or flu.

"I've had a fever on and off for the last two weeks, and a runny nose," one woman told Kelly halfway through the second day of counseling. "I just want to know: If I had anthrax, would I be dead by now?"

Kelly said yes, she would.

Later in the day, a group of custodial workers came in for handouts and explanations. "My wife won't let me sleep in the bed with her," one of them said. "She says I might give her anthrax."

"Well, sir," Kelly said, "She's going to have to come up with a new excuse."

By that night, investigators found what they believed to be the source of O'Connor's exposure: a handwritten letter, dated September 18, that had been postmarked in Trenton, New Jersey, across the Hudson River. It was almost identical to a letter found at the *New York Post,* addressed to the paper's editor. That letter was also postmarked Trenton, September 18.

On October 15, in Washington, D.C., an intern in the Capitol Hill office of Senate Majority Leader Tom Daschle cut open a hand-printed envelope, taped along its edges, that released a puff of white powder. It was postmarked October 9. It had been mailed in Trenton.

———

The ring of a telephone jolted Scott Harper out of a deep sleep. He fumbled for the bedside clock on the hotel nightstand. It was after 3:00 a.m.

"Good morning, Dr. Harper," said Hamilton's voice. "This is your wake-up call."

It was less than eighteen hours since the letter from Trenton was opened in Daschle's office. Preliminary tests at the scene suggested the powder it contained was anthrax. Now a late-night test at USAM-RIID, the government's chief lab for biological defense research, had confirmed the powder's identity and established that it was qualitatively different, finer and more expertly made, than the material recovered from the letters sent to New York. In Atlanta, a team of senior scientists had been wakened by middle-of-the-night phone calls telling them to be on a chartered plane at 6:00 a.m. One of those phone calls had jarred Hamilton awake as well. He pored over lists of EIS members, trying to sort out who was still doing World Trade Center follow-up, or at the anthrax investigations in New York and Florida. He found Scott's name. Scott was not at any of the investigations; he had been given a week off in Washington, to take a review course for his board certification exams in infectious disease. It was his second try at the course. On his first attempt, he had been yanked away to work on an outbreak of Ebola in Uganda.

He was not going to finish the course the second time, either. Hamilton told him to get up, check out, and meet the CDC team by 9:00 a.m. They would be setting up emergency investigation space in the D.C. Health Department behind Union Station, a ten-minute walk from Capitol Hill.

Because of the New York cases, Hill staff had gotten hastily drafted training on how to handle suspicious pieces of mail. The intern who opened the letter sent to Daschle did as she had been trained: She laid the letter on the floor and called the U.S. Capitol Police, who got to the office within five minutes and confirmed that the powder was anthrax before a half-hour had passed. Daschle's office was a two-story suite that stretched from the fifth to the sixth floor of the Hart Senate Office Building. The powder in the envelope, so finely milled that it could barely be seen, spread rapidly through both floors, aided by a ventilation system that was not turned off until 10:30 a.m. The scene was chaotic. FBI agents, first responders, and staff from the office of the Capitol's physician piled into the suite and a matching one next door that belonged to Senator Russell Feingold, swabbing surfaces and handing out emergency three-day packets of antibiotics to anyone who had been nearby. Staff were herded up to the ninth floor by first responders to be swabbed and tested, and then led back to the office suites' sixth-floor entrances, before they were let go for the day at 3:00 p.m. More than four hundred people in the two offices had been exposed to the powder.

The anxiety that had been caused by the New York letters increased exponentially. Those had targeted members of the media elite, though the effects had fallen not on anchors and editors but on lower-level staff. This letter struck at the heart of the government, though with Daschle out of his office that morning, it also did not reach its intended target.

The CDC team reached the Hart Building barely twenty-four hours after the letter was opened. They needed to establish as quickly as possible where the powder had spread and who had been placed at risk. The southwest quadrant of the building where the offices lay had been closed. By the end of the day, the rest of the building would be also. The Capitol physician had offered nasal swabbing and emergency doses of antibiotics to anyone in the building who felt at risk from the powder. Over three days, 2,172 people lined up, including six law enforcement members who went into Daschle's office without putting on protective equipment first.

"We needed to get just the basic epidemiology at first," Scott said. "What did this complex look like? The person who opened the letter, where had she been sitting? Who else was working nearby? We spent a lot of time talking to the CDC to determine what the best advice was to give these people—there was so little data about exposures like this—and a lot of time talking to the staff themselves, trying to answer their questions."

The pressure was intense. Mail delivery stopped throughout the Capitol for fear of other letters that might be lurking. Tours stopped. On October 17, the House of Representatives voted itself out of session and shut down. The Senate pointedly remained in session, though it closed two more buildings temporarily for testing.

Between Trenton and the Capitol, the Daschle letter had passed through the Washington, D.C., Postal Processing and Distribution Center, commonly known as the Brentwood facility. Almost all mail posted or received in Washington passed through Brentwood. Because the Daschle letter had been sealed with tape on all its seams, the CDC thought no anthrax could have escaped along its route through the postal system. The Postal Service, disinclined to shut down such a huge facility, agreed. On October 18, events challenged that decision. Early that morning, the CDC's lab in Atlanta confirmed two cases of cutaneous anthrax in workers at the New Jersey processing center where both sets of letters had been postmarked. In response, the New Jersey Department of Health and Senior Services shut the postal center down.

Two days later, the assumption that postal workers were in no danger was shattered. A doctor at Inova Fairfax Hospital in northern Virginia called the CDC's anthrax hotline with a report of a patient who was severely ill with inhalational anthrax. He was a fifty-six-year-old man named Leroy Richmond. He worked at the Brentwood center.

———

Richmond was conscious. Scott was hurriedly dispatched to interview him. The FBI beat him to the hospital, and they stayed by Richmond's bedside while Scott examined him. He was a big man, a nonsmoker who had previously been healthy. For several days, he had been feeling as though he had the flu, with chills and fever, nausea and night sweats. When he arrived at the emergency department the previous evening, he had looked only slightly ill; he had some shortness of breath and a fast heart rate, but his temperature and blood work were normal, and the doctors who saw him noticed nothing seriously amiss. A chest X-ray and a CAT scan changed their minds. The tests showed a widened mediastinum, enlarged lymph nodes, and fluid in both lungs. Now he was feverish, coughing up phlegm and having difficulty speaking. But he was awake and alert, though the toxins produced by the anthrax bacteria were wreaking havoc in his system.

Scott talked to Richmond about how he had been feeling. He went over the past twelve hours with Susan Bersoff-Matcha, the attending physician, and Thom Mayer, the emergency department chief. He studied the X-rays and the CAT scan images, noting the opaque areas where the lymph nodes in the center of Richmond's chest were filling with blood and dissolving as the tissue died. Finally, he checked a culture of Richmond's blood that the ER had started the night before. It had been cooking long enough for bacteria to grow, if there were any. Under the microscope, the culture revealed the distinctive long chains of B. anthracis.

The Fairfax doctors had done good work, but the CDC needed to confirm the diagnosis. Scott took a series of swabs and samples from Richmond and packed them with blue ice into a Styrofoam container. He had to get the samples to a borrowed corporate jet that was landing in an hour. The FBI summoned a Virginia state trooper for him.

"I got in the car, and said to the driver—a big guy, stoic, early twenties, maybe—'You know what this is, right?' " Scott said. "And he said, 'Oh, yeah. Do you want the light and sirens on?' I didn't think that was necessary. He did though. So we raced, lights blazing and sirens blaring, all the way to the airport."

The jet the CDC had borrowed had brought more staff members from Atlanta. The team, which had started out with eleven members, now numbered more than twenty. They were needed. The day Scott visited Fairfax, one of Richmond's co-workers, also fifty-six, checked into the same hospital with similar symptoms: three days of headache, chills, low fever, and nausea, followed by drenching sweats and a cough. Chest X-ray and CAT scan showed similar findings to Richmond's case—widened mediastinum, engorged lymph nodes, fluid collecting in the lining of the lungs—and anthrax bacteria grew from the man's blood.

Early the next morning, October 21, the CDC's Atlanta labs called with the results of the tests from the samples Scott had rushed to the airplane. Richmond incontrovertibly had inhalational anthrax. Faced with confirmation that bacteria had somehow leaked from a sealed letter, the CDC changed its recommendations: Everyone who worked in the Brentwood center should be checked for exposure and put on antibiotics to short-circuit any developing infection. The postal service agreed. Brentwood was shut.

It was too late. At 8:45 that night, Brentwood worker Thomas Morris Jr., fifty-five, died at Greater Southeast Community Hospital in Washington, less than fifteen hours after he called 911. At 9:30 the next morning, Brentwood worker Joseph Curseen, forty-seven, died at Southern Maryland Hospital Center, six hours after collapsing in his bathroom at home. They were the second and third fatalities of the anthrax attacks, but not the last.

———

Brentwood had more than 2,400 employees. It was 500,000 square feet in size. More than 60 million pieces of mail had gone through its high-speed sorting machines since the Daschle letter passed through on October 11. Health authorities had no way to predict how far the letter's contamination might have spread. Every person, machine, and working area in the center would have to be checked.

The CDC deployment expanded and expanded again, from twenty to thirty to approximately eighty. They spread out across an entire floor of the D.C. health department, crammed into borrowed offices, cubicles, and conference rooms. The center of the encampment was a windowless "situation room," a training classroom that came pre-stocked with computers and now was strewn with phones, whiteboards, charging cradles for phones and PDAs, and empty Power Bar wrappers. Taped to the walls were handwritten posters listing temporary computer passwords, cell phone numbers, and contacts at every local health department and the forty-nine major hospitals in the local area. A scrawled note pinned to one wall instructed: "Shred everything."

The group divided into teams: surveillance, to search public health labs and intensive care units for leads on possible new cases; epidemiology, tracking the post office and political workers who might have been exposed; the environmental team, supervising the sampling and cleanup of the Capitol Hill buildings, Brentwood and subsidiary post offices; a group handling relationships with the postal service; another group simply to keep track of the thousands of biological and environmental samples shipped to the CDC and to other labs that had agreed to help. Finally, there was the clinical investigations team, ten epidemiologists including Scott, his EIS classmate Kip Baggett, and former EIS officer Scott Fridkin. They were building a database of every recognized and suspected case of anthrax, cutaneous and inhalational, and everything that could be found out about them: what their exposure might have been, how long their incubation period lasted, which symptoms showed first and turned out to be most serious, what tests their doctors had performed.

There were more than enough cases to keep them busy. By the day Curseen died, nineteen people in several states had developed symptoms that would later prove to be inhalational or cutaneous anthrax. Many more—members of the worried well who had never been near an anthrax spore—had reported themselves to private doctors; they needed to be checked and tested, just in case.

The teams' leaders met every morning at 7:30. The entire group met twelve hours later to share each team's findings with all the others. Afterward, they went back to work again, usually until about midnight. Twice a day, after the morning meeting and before the close of the business day, Scott's team performed what they called "running the list": taking every lead they had gathered from the surveillance team or the CDC hotline and checking with doctors, hospitals, and health departments for updates. Late one afternoon in late October, the clinical team hunched around a speakerphone one cubicle away from where they had plugged in their laptops.

"We have the wife of a postal worker. Her blood and urine cultures are negative," said the voice on the other end, a staff member at the Maryland Department of Health and Mental Hygiene in Baltimore.

Fridkin, who had been following that case, scribbled the results on a legal pad. "We think this is a low-probability exposure," he said.

"We have a woman with flu-like symptoms and a negative culture," the official continued.

"We can classify her as no apparent disease," said Dr. John Jernigan, the team leader.

"We have a post office worker with a rash on the forehead and an ulcerated ear lobe," the health department representative said. "Johns Hopkins University doctors cannot rule out anthrax."

The CDC group fell silent. It was more than a week since the deaths, and the rate at which they were discovering real cases of anthrax had slowed dramatically, but they remained uneasy. None of them could forget that the Brentwood cases had taken the CDC by surprise. They did not feel responsible for the deaths—they thought the recommendations on how to handle Brentwood had been made on the best science available at the time—but they were determined that there should be no more.

The next day, Scott went up to Baltimore, to view photographs and lab results from Curseen's autopsy. He did not mind post-mortems; his father was a pathologist who had brought interesting bits of tissue home to show him, and he had had a summer job in a pathology lab. Still, the experience left him somber.

"Because this is, really, a homicide," he said a few hours afterward. "And because usually in an outbreak, when you see three or four or five of something, you know that's the tip of the iceberg. And we have three deaths so far."

The pressure to prevent any more fatalities was relentless. Kelly Moore joined the still-expanding team on October 23. She was assigned to helping to educate the postal workers, and to tracking down the employees of government agency mailrooms who might not have heard of the Brentwood closure. On her way out of the health department one morning, her supervisor stopped her.

"Kelly," she said, "your job today is to make sure that no one else from Brentwood dies."

The known effects of the anthrax attacks came to a close on November 21, with the death of a ninety-four-year-old Connecticut retiree named Ottilie Lundgren. She was the twenty-second person known to have been infected in the letter attacks, and the fifth to die of inhalational anthrax, after Stevens, Morris and Curseen, and Kathy Nguyen, a sixty-one-year-old hospital worker in Manhattan. Nguyen and Lundgren's deaths were provisionally attributed to anthrax contamination on the surface of their mail, but a source for the anthrax spores that killed them has never been found.

The remaining seventeen victims—eleven with cutaneous anthrax and six others with the inhalational form—recovered from the disease, though some continue to experience long-term health problems.

The presumed first letter in the attacks, which must have arrived sometime in mid-September at the office where Bob Stevens worked, was never found. The last known anthrax-loaded letter was discovered November 16, in a barrel of Capitol Hill mail that had been quarantined October 17. It was addressed to Senator Patrick Leahy. According to analysts at the CDC and the Department of Defense, the anthrax loaded into the letters became progressively more refined as the mailings continued, as though its creator were increasing his or her expertise with practice, or as a message.

The creator of the anthrax, and presumed perpetrator of the attacks, has never been identified.

More than two thousand members of the CDC's staff worked on the Trade Center attacks and the anthrax letters. Of the 146 first- and second-year EIS members, 136 of them—everyone who was able to travel and had not been inadvertently trapped in an overseas posting—went to one of the crisis sites. More than forty of them went out at least twice; more than a handful went four or five times. By the end of the year, most were back at their normal jobs, many with their perspectives permanently altered.

"There was so much going on, and it happened so quickly," Scott said. "I came to realize that's how things work in public health: When there is a big crisis, you make the best decisions you can, usually with limited data."

"The enormity of the task was so incredible that we didn't have time to mourn, or to react the way we would have had we been sitting on the sidelines," Kelly said. "But I'm glad I wasn't on the sidelines. There wasn't much time to think, but I remember very clearly thinking that we were involved in making history."

THIRTEEN

SARS

March–July 2003,
Hanoi and Bangkok

JOEL MONTGOMERY PULLED THE TRAYS that had been set aside for him out of the lab refrigerator, and winced. The trays were full of plastic bags. The bags were full of tubes of blood, labeled with the names of patients and the dates the blood had been drawn from their veins. Some of the tubes had popped open, and the blood inside them had pooled and clotted in the bottom of the bags. The labels had soaked up the blood, and some of them had slipped free of the tubes they were meant to identify. There were almost thirty bags, and more than eight hundred tubes of blood.

The tubes were resting inside a refrigerator in a high-ceilinged, marble-floored laboratory at the National Institute of Hygiene and Epidemiology in Hanoi. They represented a day-by-day record of what had gone on inside the bodies of the first group of people recognized as victims of severe acute respiratory syndrome. The blood in the tubes contained valuable information that could help the CDC understand how the virus that caused SARS evaded the immune system, and how the disease progressed.

The EIS had shipped Joel to Hanoi to help get that information. The blood had to be extracted from the tubes, spun down for its serum, divided into fractions, and shipped off to laboratories that had the facilities to analyze it safely and fast. The need for data was urgent. It was late March. The disease had been leaping around the globe for more than a month, but it had been detected and named only two weeks earlier, and the virus that caused it had been identified only four days ago. Worldwide, more than 1,300 people were known to be ill. Here in Vietnam, three nurses and a doctor were dead, fifty-five of their colleagues and relatives were hospitalized, and the hospital where they had all worked had locked its doors with its sick staff still inside. It was the hospital staff's blood that lay in the refrigerated tubes.

There was no way of knowing at this point how much virus the blood contained, or how hazardous exposure to it might be. Joel slid a Tyvek hood over his head and settled the seal of its faceplate around the bones of his jaw and cheeks. He switched on the motor of the air supply, took a deep breath, and got to work.

———

Johnny Chen was very sick, and none of the health workers treating him were quite sure why.

It was the morning of March 3, a Monday. It was early, but Hanoi is a town that rises early. The neighborhood loudspeakers that play inspirational music and scold residents for littering had crackled to life before 6:00 a.m. Dr. Vu Hoang Thu, a forty-three-year-old internist, had downed a small cup of dark filtered coffee and left the house she shared with her husband and two teenage sons before the sun pierced between the tree trunks in Lenin Park in the center of town. She was at the French Hospital, a rounded, blocky building of pink and white stucco that lay across a wide boulevard from the park, before the nurses on the night shift handed off the care of their patients to the staff coming in for the day.

Vu was one of the physicians assigned to the fifty-six-bed hospital's general medical ward. Chen was one of her patients. The forty-seven-year-old American had been at the hospital for almost a week. He had checked himself in the previous Wednesday, choosing the small private institution over the sprawling, scruffy campus of state-run Bach Mai Hospital next door. He was a businessman, based in China, so he could afford the French Hospital. He had started to feel sick, with a high fever and a puzzling fatigue, immediately after arriving from Hong Kong two days before.

Slowly but steadily, Chen had gotten worse. Despite antipyretics, his fever had stayed stubbornly high. Despite antibiotics, his lungs were slowly filling with fluid; on X-rays, Vu could see the opaque shadow of inflammation moving slowly up his chest. A blood test suggested he might be infected with influenza B, the influenza virus variety that was most common in Asia; influenza B was a milder variety than influenza A, which caused wide-ranging epidemics in the Northern Hemisphere most winters. Based on the influenza test result, the staff had given him an antiviral drug, but there was no sign it had helped. On Saturday he started to cough explosively. On Sunday morning, he slipped into severe respiratory distress. He was lethargic and having trouble breathing. His skin had a greyish tinge, and when he tried to speak, he made no sense.

Clearly he was not getting enough oxygen. Vu ordered Chen put on a ventilator. It was a quick process when it went smoothly, but it was always tense. It was easy to make a mistake, and a doctor had to go nose-to-nose with the patient to sight clearly down the airway. This intubation had gone well. One nurse sedated Chen and gave him an injection that briefly paralyzed him. Another stood by his shoulder, pressing down on his throat cartilage to close his esophagus so the tube would not go the wrong way. A doctor slid the curved laryngoscope into his mouth, squinting down its sights and easing the tube along its guiding stylet, down his throat and between his vocal cords. Within moments, Chen was hooked to the ventilator. Almost immediately, his color began to improve.

That had been the day before. So when she reached the hospital, Vu was surprised to find that Chen was no better: The machine was supplying him with oxygen, but he was still obviously severely ill. There was another surprise awaiting her. One of the nurses who had assisted with his intubation was tired and had a high fever, and she was beginning to cough.

———

All over Asia that month, doctors were concerned about influenza.

One week before Chen checked into the French Hospital, the government of Hong Kong announced that two members of a local family were infected with a strain of influenza known as H5N1. The father of the family, thirty-three-year-old Ko Yan-Kit, had died in Hong Kong's Princess Margaret Hospital on February 16. Ko's wife, ten-year-old daughter, nine-year-old son, and father were also ill. Their youngest child, eight-year-old Mei-ling, was dead; she had died of pneumonia February 4, during a family visit to a small town in Fujian province north of Hong Kong.

There were two worrisome pieces of news in the family's misfortune. The first was the presence of H5N1. It was a strain of influenza A, the most common of the three types of flu virus, but it was not a strain that was supposed to show up in people. In the decades since 1933, when the flu virus was identified, research had shown that there were fifteen subtypes of influenza A, but that humans caught only three of them: H1, H2, and H3. (The H stood for hemagglutinin, a protein on the surface of the virus; the N that followed after it stood for neuraminidase, a second surface protein.)

H5N1, the strain found in the Ko family, was a disease of chickens. It was an ugly disease. It was also called "highly pathogenic avian influenza," and it deserved the name: It was fast-moving and fatal and could destroy a flock in days. An influenza expert had once described it as "chicken Ebola." H5N1 was not supposed to infect people, but it had at least once before. In the fall of 1997, it jumped species, infecting eighteen people in Hong Kong and killing six of them before the local government slaughtered every chicken in the territory and shut the outbreak down.

The episode had shaken world health authorities, and not just because it had killed one out of every three victims. Flu experts lived in terror of a new strain of the virus, one that would sweep the world in a global pandemic. The "Spanish" flu of 1918 had done that, and left 40 million dead in its wake. And a strain that jumped from another species was as novel as could be imagined. Human immune systems would have no protection against it, and existing vaccines would have no power to stop it.

The second piece of bad news was the probable location of the Ko family's infection. They were likely, based on the usual incubation period of flu, to have acquired the disease while visiting relatives in Fujian. It was a setting to make a flu scientist shudder. Outside its main city, Xiamen, much of Fujian is rural and agricultural, full of small villages where residents keep a pig and a few chickens or perhaps some ducks. By a quirk of biology, pigs are vulnerable not only to the influenza viruses specific to swine, but to human and bird flu viruses as well. If a pig is infected by several subtypes of influenza at once, the viruses can swap genes, potentially producing a novel flu strain that carries the lethality of avian influenza and the contagiousness of human flu.

Over the years, researchers had noted that most of the world's new flu strains originated in southern China, and they feared the potential of China's backyard agriculture to brew even more new viruses. If the Ko family had been infected in Fujian and had brought the virus back to Hong Kong, the implications were grave indeed.

———

The concerns about influenza were not limited to Hong Kong.

The previous November, a puzzling respiratory illness had started cropping up in Guangdong, the province south of Fujian. Guangdong wraps around Hong Kong on three sides, and its border with the territory is porous because the province, and especially its capital Guangzhou, is the fervent center of China's new capitalism. Guangzhou holds more than 5 million people. Its downtown is a maze of skyscraper construction, even though the near outskirts are as humble as the villages in Fujian.

The cases of illness started in Foshan, a fast-growing town of more than 3 million that lies southwest of Guangzhou. Week by week, the unexplained pneumonia spread through the countryside of the Pearl River Delta. The stories that appeared in the state-run newspapers—in Zhongshan, south of Guangzhou, and Heyuan, north of the city—denied the outbreak's existence so vociferously that they effectively confirmed its existence. Rumors that health care workers were sick became so common that the World Health Organization asked the Chinese Ministry of Health to comment. The reply that came back by email said there was only a minor outbreak of influenza B.

On February 3, a forty-year-old man checked himself into the No. 2 Hospital in Guangzhou. His lungs were filling up from pneumonia and he was coughing and feverish. The illness spread rapidly through the hospital. Within two weeks, there were enough health care workers sick with the same unexplained ailment to fill an entire ward. The remaining staff were frantic. They worked long hours, trading back and forth between their sick colleagues and the steady flow of patients coming in from outside.

By the second week of February, the rumor of the outbreak had reached a new audience: the Internet. In a chat room on a site called Teachers.net, a California fourth-grade teacher named Catherine Strommen received a note from a Guangzhou teacher she had spoken with a few times before. The note asked: "Have you heard of the terrible sickness in my city?"

She had not, but she thought she knew someone who might. Strommen's husband had been in the Navy, and they had once been assigned to Hawaii where they made friends with a Navy physician and epidemiologist who lived nearby. The neighbor, Dr. Stephen O. Cunnion, was now an international health consultant in suburban Washington. He relayed her question to ProMED, a listserv for reporting disease outbreaks that is run by the International Society for Infectious Diseases and has more than thirty thousand subscribers worldwide.

After vetting by the moderators, Cunnion's post appeared the next day, February 10. It quoted Strommen's note: " 'Have you heard of an epidemic in Guangzhou? An acquaintance of mine . . . lives there and reports that the hospitals there have been closed and people are dying.'"

Cunnion got dozens of replies, though none from China. But less than a day later, the Guangdong Department of Health made its first official statement about the outbreak.

Yes, the agency said, there had been an outbreak of about three hundred cases of pneumonia and five deaths, but it was ending.

In fact, it was not ending, though no one outside China would learn that for six more weeks. It had spread to at least eight cities within Guangdong. At the No. 2 Hospital, more than fifty health care workers were sick, and their healthy colleagues were growing exhausted caring for them. One of the healthy ones was Dr. Liu Jian-Lun, a sixty-four-year-old professor of medicine at Zhongshan University in Guangzhou. In late February, he took a break from the epidemic. His nephew was getting married in Hong Kong, and Dr. Liu wanted to be there—even though, in the past few days, he had been starting to feel a little unwell.

On February 21, Dr. Liu and his wife checked into the Metropole Hotel in Kowloon, on the mainland side of Hong Kong. They were given room 911. On the ninth floor with them were a random group of travelers whose names, or fates at least, would soon become known worldwide. One of them was Johnny Chen.

———

The French Hospital, where Chen arrived five days after spending the night on the same hotel floor as Liu—whether they ever met, or even passed in the hall, has never been established—had become the site of a ferocious outbreak. By March 5, three days after Chen's intubation, the nurse who had helped grew so sick that she was hospitalized. By March 6, nine more of the staff had the same symptoms that she did: sudden high fever, deep malaise, nonproductive cough.

"From the fifth, we did blood tests every day, for the entire staff," Vu said. "We didn't find anything."

The medical staff had heard of the influenza cases in Hong Kong and the pneumonia epidemic on the mainland. They knew Chen had passed through Hong Kong, and they suspected he had acquired his illness there. The hospital's management called the local WHO office to let them know that something inexplicable might have crossed the border. WHO has only a small group in Hanoi, headed by an elegant Frenchwoman named Pascale Brudon. She asked a member of her staff, Dr. Carlo Urbani, to take a look.

Urbani was forty-six, a big, cheerful man with dark hair and a wide forehead who came from Castelplanio, a small town on Italy's Adriatic coast. He had spent much of his medical life in Africa and Asia, and he had come to Vietnam with his wife and three children to work on programs preventing parasitic diseases in children. He was the former president of the Italian branch of *Médecins Sans frontières,* known in the United States as Doctors Without Borders, and had helped accept the Nobel Peace Prize given to the group in 1999.

"Health and dignity are indissociable in human beings," he said at the ceremony. "It is a duty to stay close to victims and guarantee their rights."

Urbani made his first visit to the French Hospital on February 28, two days after Chen was admitted. Like the hospital staff, he had heard the news from Hong Kong, and he worried that Chen might have carried avian influenza into Vietnam. He was especially struck that health care workers were falling ill so quickly. On March 5, he sent a warning email to the WHO's communicable diseases division in Geneva, and he began coming to the French Hospital every day, sometimes twice a day. He began to worry the disease was not influenza. He kept checking the sick staff, swabbing their throats for analysis and drawing their blood, looking for a clue that would explain what was making them so ill.

Chen's family had him medevaced to Hong Kong on March 6. His departure came too late for the French Hospital. On the 7th, two more cases developed, making twelve in all, and Urbani recommended the hospital isolate its sick staff in one ward on its second floor. On the 8th, five of the twelve developed bilateral pneumonia. Urbani herded the remaining staff into the cafeteria and urged them all to wear whatever protective gear the hospital had in stock, especially face masks, at all times. On the 9th, there were fifteen cases. In a desperate bid to halt the disease's advance, the hospital turned off its air-conditioning.

On March 11, several things happened at once. The count of sick doctors and nurses rose to thirty-five; four of their family members were ill as well. The hospital did not have enough staff left to operate—it barely had enough to care for its own sick personnel—and so it closed its doors. Its patients were transferred to Bach Mai Hospital next door. The sick staff, most of them now gasping with pneumonia or sedated and on ventilators, stayed behind. They were accidental victims of a still-unidentified plague, and their workplace had become a plague hospital.

Inexplicably, Vu was not sick. When the hospital sealed its doors, she remained inside. She would not come out for more than three weeks.

"I stayed for my colleagues," she said. "I said to the others who were not sick that we should try to continue. But we were very worried, very scared."

On the same day, Urbani made a morning visit to the hospital, to check on the sick staff and take another set of samples. Then he hurried back to the WHO office. He was due in Bangkok that evening; he was giving a talk at a scientific meeting, a long-standing commitment, the next day.

From the airport, he called Brudon.

"He said he was not feeling very well," she said. "He said, Pascale, I think I have got this disease."

———

Urbani's first alarmed communiqué to the WHO about Chen had been shared with the CDC. So had subsequent accounts that he sent over the ensuing ten days, describing the clinical features of the health care workers' cases and the epidemiology he had pieced together of how they became infected.

He had reported Chen's illness, at first, as a suspected case of influenza—either the avian influenza that had appeared in Hong Kong, or the influenza B that Vietnam had found in its earliest tests on Chen. The reports came into a flu office that was already on guard against the bird flu. Dr. Keiji Fukuda, the CDC's chief of influenza epidemiology and its in-house expert on avian influenza, was in Beijing at the Chinese government's invitation, ready to search for any links between the new H5N1 cases and the Guangdong epidemic. The invitation had reportedly been issued only after HHS Secretary Tommy Thompson applied polite pressure to his Chinese counterpart, the minister of health. There was certainly no evidence of an enthusiastic welcome within China: Fukuda and his WHO colleagues had been in Beijing for two weeks, but had not yet received permission from the Guangdong health department to travel there.

Urbani's notes were being read as well by Tim Uyeki, who had joined the flu branch as an EIS officer in 1998 and stayed to be a staff epidemiologist when his two years were up. Uyeki was a pediatrician, trained in Cleveland and California, who had a public policy degree as well as the standard M.D./M.P.H. combination shared by most of the CDC's physicians.

"Between the incubation period and some of the other clinical features Urbani described, we didn't think it sounded like influenza," Uyeki said. "Especially if it was influenza B, because B doesn't cause severe outbreaks. If it was influenza B, it would have been the most severe influenza B virus in world history."

The puzzle of which pathogen lay at the heart of the outbreak increased the CDC's desire to get to Vietnam to help. But there was a hurdle in the way: It had to be asked. The investigation belonged to the WHO, and the decision to allow the WHO to bring in extra investigators rested with the Vietnamese Ministry of Health. The WHO's relationship to countries is like the CDC's to the states. It has abundant influence but little overt power; it can persuade, but not compel. On March 9, the ministry's permission arrived: It would allow the WHO to bring in two more investigators. The WHO elected to send Dr. Hitoshi Oshitani, the communicable diseases expert in its Western Pacific office, based in Manila. The CDC sent Tim Uyeki.

There was no time to get a visa. Uyeki left immediately, carting three trunks of medical supplies as well as his own bags. He headed for Bangkok, because he could enter Thailand without advance permission and because the staff there, the largest CDC group in Asia, needed to be warned of what was going on. Bangkok is a tourism crossroads, but it is also a medical hub for most of Southeast Asia. In Atlanta, the CDC's planners could envision a scenario in which a member of Asia's new super-rich was attacked by the mystery pneumonia and fled to Bangkok for care, spreading the disease to yet another country. And if the situation in Vietnam got worse, the CDC workers in Bangkok might be recruited to help.

It was very early March 11 by the time Uyeki reached Bangkok. He fought his way through the city's gridlock to Scott Dowell's office in Nonthaburi, a suburb embedded in the city's northward sprawl. In a tense meeting, Uyeki described the explosive outbreak in the French Hospital, and the little the CDC knew so far about the epidemic in Guangdong. It was eight years since the Rwandan refugee crisis, and Dowell was now chief of the Bangkok office of the International Emerging Infections Program, a group that the CDC was gradually deploying around the world as an early-warning system for unusual diseases. He had set up the office, the first one in the program, in fall 2001. After eighteen months in Thailand, he had a vivid appreciation of how quickly a new organism could take root there.

Dowell thought the Hanoi WHO representative, Bjorn Melgaard, needed to hear Uyeki's report as well. But time was short: Uyeki was leaving on an evening flight, and he still needed a Vietnamese visa and several more boxes of supplies. Melgaard squeezed them into his schedule over lunch, and listened somberly as Uyeki described CDC's concerns about the Vietnamese and Chinese outbreaks. They discussed, briefly and apprehensively, the strategies they would have to deploy if a case of the disease landed in Bangkok. Then Dowell rushed Uyeki off again.

Uyeki landed in Bangkok at about 8:00 p.m. and argued his trunks of supplies through customs. That took more than an hour. He found a taxi to take him the thirty-minute ride into the city, and went straight to the WHO office, a cream-colored modernized villa on a busy street not far from the architectural wedding cake of Hanoi's Opera House. He had expected to meet Urbani there, but the villa was dark, and the gates were locked. He had no way of knowing that he and Urbani had passed, literally, in mid-air.

At about the same time, in Bangkok, Melgaard called Dowell at home.

"What we discussed this afternoon has happened," he said. "And it is worse than you imagined. It is one of our staff."

The next morning, for the first time in ten years, the WHO issued a global alert.

———

It came too late. While the CDC and the WHO had been focused on Hanoi, the still-unexplained disease had seeded itself around the world.

On the afternoon that Dr. Liu checked into the Metropole Hotel, a Chinese-Canadian family were checking out. They lived outside Toronto, but they had been visiting their son in Hong Kong for the celebration of the Lunar New Year. They arrived home February 23. A few days later, Kwan Sui Chu, the seventy-eight-year-old mother of the family, began to feel feverish. On March 5, she died at home of a heart attack. Two days later, her son Tse Chi Kwai, felt feverish too. He sought help in the crowded emergency department of Scarborough Grace Hospital in a Toronto suburb.

Tse died March 13. His visit to the hospital started a chain of infection that would produce 251 cases of illness in Canada, and forty-three deaths.

Staying on the same floor as Dr. Liu were three young women from Singapore who had come to Hong Kong on a shopping trip. When they returned home, they sparked an outbreak that sickened thirty-four others. A Singaporean doctor who treated some of the first patients infected by the women visited New York City for a medical meeting, and then flew home through Europe. He was taken off the plane in Frankfurt, along with his pregnant wife and mother-in-law, and hospitalized there, becoming Europe's first cases of the new disease.

On the night that Dr. Liu stayed in the hotel, he attended his nephew's wedding banquet. He infected one of the other relatives there, as well as a local resident who was visiting the hotel. Both men were treated at separate Hong Kong hospitals. A visitor to one of the hospitals later took a plane to Beijing, carrying the infection into China's interior and passing it to travelers who brought it to Inner Mongolia and Taiwan.

Dr. Liu checked himself into a Hong Kong hospital on February 22. He warned the staff to put him in isolation, and he told some of them about the epidemic he had helped to treat in Guangdong. He died March 4. Thanks to Liu's visit, and an unknown number of other patients who may have crossed the border, there would eventually be 1,755 cases of the disease and 299 deaths in Hong Kong.

One of those was Johnny Chen. He died in a Hong Kong hospital on March 13, one week after being medevac'd from Hanoi.

It would take weeks for those connections to emerge. Meanwhile, in Hanoi, one of the nurses who had treated Chen died March 15. The doctor who intubated him died March 19. Fifty-six health care workers and their families were sick, at the French Hospital and at Bach Mai. The CDC and WHO were just beginning to understand the scope of what they faced.

"What was going on in that hospital was the same thing that was going on in Guangdong province, though we had no idea what it was," Uyeki said. "It was not just a problem for Vietnam. It was a regional problem, and a global problem."

The French Hospital outbreak was not the earliest outbreak of the new illness, but it was the first to come to the world's attention, and it was the only one that had been detected and recorded from the very first case. Starting with Chen, Vu and her colleagues had collected every scrap of clinical data that might help them understand the vicious pneumonia: throat swabs, blood samples, records of vital signs, relationships between the sick, accounts of the progression of symptoms. It was all sitting in medical charts and lab refrigerators; no one had analyzed any of it, because no one had the time.

Staring at the records, Uyeki realized that it was a potential treasure trove of critically needed information. It would need a particular kind of scientist to unlock it, though: not only an epidemiologist, but a microbiologist as well. He thought about the EIS officers he had met. Then he composed an email, asking the CDC to send Joel Montgomery.

———

The CDC that received Urbani's warnings was a different agency from the one that had scrambled to respond to anthrax seventeen months before. The attacks had shaken the CDC profoundly. It had been harshly criticized in the media and in congressional hearings for allowing the Brentwood post office to remain open, exposing thousands of workers and some of its own investigators to the spores squeezed out of the letters by the machinery and causing two of the five deaths. The criticism was partially unjust—the decision had been made in concert with the U.S. Postal Service and without full knowledge of FBI and UAMRIID findings about the quality of the spores—but it had stuck. It had deeply wounded the staff. And it had produced aftereffects. CDC director Jeffrey P. Koplan, who had been at the agency with one four-year break since working on smallpox in 1972, resigned at the end of March 2002. He moved to a senior position at Emory University School of Medicine, next door to the CDC. It was a logical move, and a good job; but within the national public health community, where he was widely liked, he was thought to have sacrificed his career in a bid to draw the pressure of the attacks' aftermath away from the CDC. His departure left agency veterans demoralized, imagining political interference to come.

His replacement was Julie L. Gerberding, an infectious-disease physician and HIV scientist who had joined the CDC only four years before. Gerberding had spent her career at University of California, San Francisco, where she did some of the earliest research on the threat posed to health workers by HIV. She had come to the CDC to head its Division of Healthcare Quality and Promotion, which worked on medical errors and infections occurring inside health care institutions. In early September 2002, she had agreed to take a four-month stint as acting deputy director of the National Center for Infectious Diseases, the historic heart of the CDC. The serendipity of the temporary posting put her on the short list of CDC managers—along with Koplan, deputy director for science Dr. David Fleming, and NCID chief Dr. James M. Hughes—who were regularly put in front of the media during the chaotic aftermath of the attacks.

To the slight surprise of the agency rank and file, she turned out to be very good at it. She was distinctive-looking, with a forelock of white hair slicing through a chin-length black bob, and on-camera she appeared focused but relaxed. She had been chief resident at UCSF and still retained the knack, essential to the position, for internalizing large amounts of data and switching with speed between different trains of thought. She seldom used notes when she spoke. When Koplan stepped down, HHS Secretary Tommy Thompson reached past Fleming and Hughes and selected Gerberding to be successor. It was a bold choice, since she was not a CDC lifer and supporters feared the administration would frown on her career in AIDS research, but a smart one. Gerberding was forty-six and the first woman to head the CDC. Her scientific background gave her credibility among the many agency staff who had not even met her—DHQP, the division she had headed, was a small group off to the side of the CDC's organizational chart—and after months of their feeling targeted, Thompson's emphatic backing came as a relief.

The struggle to cope with the public alarm created by the anthrax letters—and the thousands of biological and environmental samples, as well as hoax letters, collected during the investigation—had revealed that U.S. public health, the bulwark against bioterrorism, was in terrible shape. Laboratories and communications networks, at the CDC and in the states, had been deprived of significant funding for years. The strain had brought the system close to breakdown, and in one case literally to failure: Early in the anthrax crisis, a major electrical line into the CDC had sizzled out from overload, halting all lab work for twelve hours.

The federal government made up for the years of underinvestment in one lump sum: In mid-2002, Congress passed a supplemental appropriation of $1.1 billion, for the CDC and the states, specifically to prepare for bioterrorism. On the CDC side, the money went to upgrade laboratories and information technology. The agency built a secure broadband network between health departments, recruited more than one hundred university, state, and private labs into cooperative agreements to provide help in emergencies, and threw hundreds of Web pages of disease information online. Private money flowed to the CDC as well. In the midst of anthrax, the agency had needed a place to coordinate the efforts of the several hundred investigators it sent into the field; lacking anything better, staff had dragged desks and bulletin boards into Auditorium A at the front of the campus and transformed it into a jury-rigged war room. The makeshift facility so appalled Bernard Marcus, an Atlanta philanthropist who co-founded the Home Depot chain, that he personally pledged to build the CDC a real emergency operations center. ("I have grandchildren. I am concerned about their health and welfare," he said when he disclosed the gift. "I can't wait for the federal government to see to that. If I can do it, I will.")

The $3.9 million result, augmented by gifts of equipment from fifteen tech manufacturers, was completed in early March. It was a softly lit, gleaming space of wood paneling, halogen drop lights, and liquid-crystal displays. Forty workstations with ergonomic chairs and flat-panel monitors faced a dais with three desks, for the logistics chief, the shift chief, and the situation commander. Behind the dais were wide plasma screens displaying news channels and GIS maps; behind the rows of workstations, on the other side of glass walls that blanked to opaque when a switch was thrown, were conference rooms wired with broadband video and audio and linked to the war rooms at HHS in Washington and the WHO in Geneva.

The contrast between the worn 1960s-era buildings above ground and the sleek basement bunker was jarring, like walking from real life into an imagined movie-set version of it. But the EOC, as it was quickly dubbed, was an oddly soothing place to work, hushed and energetic at the same time and without outside distractions.

On March 15, WHO director-general Gro Harlem Brundtland called the emerging epidemic "a worldwide health threat." She also gave it a name: SARS, for "severe acute respiratory syndrome." Following the WHO's lead, the CDC put the new EOC into crisis mode, moving full crews of staff underground to work in shifts around the clock. The war room became the nerve center of the nascent SARS emergency. The new disease called out the EIS: In short order, members of the group were dispatched to Hanoi, Toronto, Hong Kong, and Taiwan. The rest volunteered for rotating ops-center duty, to track the emerging epidemic and to monitor their colleagues abroad and make sure that they stayed well.

———

The early betting was that SARS was caused by a virus, since none of the antibiotics tried as treatments in countries had made the slightest difference to the progression of the disease. The WHO patched together a network of eleven labs around the world to look for the organism. The CDC found it. It was a coronavirus, named for a crown of spikes on the surface of the virus that could be seen through an electron microscope. Other coronaviruses were known to cause severe disease in animals and colds in humans, but this coronavirus had never been seen before.

A few days afterward Joel Montgomery and Dan Bausch, a physician with a tropical medicine degree, landed in Hanoi. The discovery of the virus—which was still not confirmed as the cause of SARS, but was the most plausible candidate seen so far—would give their work a target.

Vietnam's CDC equivalent was the National Institute of Hygiene and Epidemiology, or NIHE, pronounced "nee hay." NIHE was based in the old Pasteur Institute, a French colonial relic named for the premier French scientist. In another French touch, its address was 1 Yersin Street, after Alexandre Yersin, the discoverer of the plague bacillus. Unlike most of his colonial colleagues, Yersin had loved Vietnam; he had married a Vietnamese woman, settled in the country, and died and was buried there. Like the other municipal structures that had survived the French withdrawal fifty years earlier, including the Opera House and the townhouses of the gallery district, the institute's exterior was made of mellow gold stucco with delicate detail. It was a long, low building of two wings centered on a wide entrance hall with a sweeping marble staircase, and topped with a bell tower. Outwardly, it resembled a school in Provence. It looked nothing like a modern laboratory.

The inside was more modern than the outside. NIHE's specialties were virology, immunology, and disease surveillance. Its scientists were well known in Asia; it frequently hosted conferences and had its own vaccine-development arm that worked on rabies, hepatitis, and Japanese encephalitis. Still, it had never been called on to help identify a brand-new disease, and it lacked most of the high-level protections that would permit safe handling of a not-yet-understood organism. In Atlanta, the Special Pathogens Branch was performing all the SARS lab work. In Hanoi, NIHE was forced to rig a makeshift hot lab. It loaned the CDC team its influenza laboratory, an open, high-ceilinged lab with marble floors and latched wood doors pierced with small, square glass panels. It was a beautiful room, but it had no modifications that would guarantee even moderate biosafety. Joel and Dan would need to tinker with equipment and protective gear to craft a compromise that felt safe.

By email, they discussed ground rules with their Special Pathogens supervisors. The virus could cause serious disease, could be transmitted through the air, and could not currently be prevented by a vaccine. Those conclusions were obvious, and they were also troubling, because they matched three of the four conditions that Special Pathogens used to classify disease organisms as highest risk. But after looking at the scope of the worldwide epidemic—forty-nine deaths so far among 1,323 known cases of illness—they could not agree that the virus posed a high likelihood of life-threatening disease. That was the fourth condition. SARS did not meet it. It was a relief, and not only for their personal comfort. Concluding that SARS was high risk would have forced them to work under the highest hot-zone level of biosafety, BSL-4—and there was no BSL-4 lab anywhere in Vietnam. Not meeting that condition meant they could drop back to BSL-3 protections. Those were challenging enough to create: They included limiting access to the lab, making sure that building air flowed into the lab and not out of it, working inside biosafety cabinets with air circulation that flowed away from the researcher, autoclaving all the lab waste, and wearing not only basic protective gear—gowns, gloves, and face protection—but contained air supplies as well. Still, they were achievable. BSL-4 would have been impossible.

The researchers might have been able to get by with less. But they were working with whole blood, and it made them wary. There was as yet no evidence that SARS could be transmitted by blood, but it was impossible to ignore the lessons of two decades of AIDS, which had drilled into lab workers that blood was the most hazardous of all crude biological samples. They agreed to full protective gear, including powered air-purifying respirators with integral face shields and hoods.

"We were spinning the blood in a centrifuge that didn't have aerosol guards, so if we broke a tube, we didn't want to aerosolize the blood and breathe it in," Joel said. "And we had a safety cabinet, but the last time it had been inspected was 2001, so we didn't know if it had proper airflow."

They set up both their laptops, and in both of them started identical databases, so they could number the samples and keep track of all the information they could glean from the blood-soaked labels. They recruited two NIHE researchers to help them, since typing with bloody gloves would be too messy. And then they started opening the bags to catalogue the eight hundred tubes.

It took a week of fifteen-hour days to catalogue the tubes and centrifuge them, and divide the usable contents into three portions: one each for the Special Pathogens Branch, the WHO's lab network, and the researchers at NIHE. The work was intense but steady; the consequences of making a mistake and breaking a tube or slitting a glove were too dire to indulge their desire to rush for a result. The BSL-3 rules limited lab access to only a few people, so they were seldom bothered. It was oddly peaceful in the big, old-fashioned room, and it was easy to lose track of the outside world—until late one weekend morning when Joel's rented cell phone buzzed.

It was news about Carlo Urbani.

———

Scott Dowell had rushed to the airport through Bangkok's twenty-four-hour traffic to meet Urbani's flight from Hanoi. By the time he arrived, it had landed. Dowell had no idea what the parasitologist looked like, but he spotted him as soon as the bus from the airplane disgorged its passengers. Urbani was taller than most of the others, but it was his expression that caught Dowell's eye: He was pale and had a grim look on his face.

Dowell and a local quarantine officer who had joined him greeted Urbani gingerly—they were careful not to shake hands—and then led him through an unused part of the airport to an out-of-the-way driveway. They were expecting to meet an ambulance, but there was no ambulance in sight. Its crew had stopped to get protective gear. Then they had gotten lost in the airport. It would take them ninety minutes to find the right door.

Dowell and Urbani arranged two plastic chairs about six feet apart—close enough to hear each other over the traffic noise, but far enough, Dowell thought, to keep the risk of infection low. They talked.

"Carlo was quiet," Dowell said. "He wasn't particularly sick; he wasn't short of breath, he wasn't coughing. Mostly he had a bit of fever, and he was scared he would get a lot worse."

The ambulance, when it arrived, took them to Bamrasnadura Hospital, a state-run facility that the ministry of health had designated as the main quarantine hospital in case an ugly disease came to Thailand. It was after 2:00 a.m. They found Urbani a room that was off by itself on the third floor, away from areas where patients were being cared for. Bamras, as it is called, is a typical tropical hospital. The wards are open to the air at both ends, and there is no air-conditioning, so there was no such thing as a negative-pressure room with one-way airflow that could keep disease organisms from floating out into the hospital. Dowell and the staff hastily improvised one, propping fans in the windows to suck air in from the hallway and blow it outside.

They moved Urbani in, and checked his vital signs. He had a fever of about 100 degrees. His chest sounded clear when they listened to it. His chest X-ray was clear as well, and the level of oxygen in his blood was acceptable.

"For the most part he was not a patient who needed to be in a hospital," Dowell said. "But he was scared, and depressed. In Hanoi he had seen patients who were well in the morning and very sick in the afternoon, and he feared it would be quick."

Dowell had been working on plans for a conference in northern Thailand. It was starting in two days. He asked Mike Martin, an internist who had come to Bangkok to work on the CDC's Asian HIV program, to take over Urbani's care.

Martin was approaching forty. He had trained in Louisville, worked in Sri Lanka and Zambia, and studied in England, getting a degree from the London School of Tropical Medicine and Hygiene, before joining the EIS in 2000. He and Dowell had met during Martin's first EIS year, when they had both been sent to work on an outbreak of Ebola hemorrhagic fever in Gulu, Uganda. The five-month outbreak had sickened 428 people and killed more than half of them, including twelve Ugandan nurses and a doctor, Matthew Lukwiya, who had become Dowell's friend.

When Dowell called Martin the day after Urbani arrived, he warned him: "This could be worse than Ebola." He meant that it appeared likely to be more infectious, though the comment suggested as well how frightening the new disease could be. Martin understood. He agreed to take the case, and he went over to Bamras to meet Urbani.

"He was well," Martin said. "He had a little low-grade fever, some muscle aches and pains, perhaps some coughing. Nothing seemed bad. We had heard about mild cases of the disease, and I figured he was one of them. I thought, Maybe this is going to be OK."

Urbani, though, was still scared, and he felt isolated in the room they had stashed him in. It was at one end of the ward, at a point where the corridor ended in a cast-concrete balcony—well away from the stairs and from other patients, but out of sight of the nurses' station or anyone else walking by. They decided to move him into the center of the floor, directly opposite the nurses. In three days, the hospital cleared the ward of patients and made the floor into an isolation suite, putting up double walls of glass that enclosed Urbani's new room and the nursing station, with a sealed one-way corridor in between. From their desk, the nurses had a clear view of Urbani in bed about eight feet away. It was a little too far, though, to see the pulse monitor and oximeter, so to read them in a hurry they kept a set of binoculars on top of the desk. To see him face-to-face required additional steps. Everyone entering the floor wore basic gear: gowns, gloves, and a fitted N-95 mask with mesh that was small enough to catch viruses before they could be inhaled. Between leaving the nursing station and entering the corridor to Urbani's room, the doctors and nurses put on an extra layer of protection: a second gown and gloves, shoe covers, and eye protection.

For more than a week, the arrangements felt like overkill. Urbani still had a low fever, and a cough that came and went. He complained of shortness of breath, and the staff put him on some supplemental oxygen, from a cannula that hung just underneath his nose. Dowell had been shipped to Taiwan, where SARS had infiltrated after being held off for weeks. He called every night to keep Urbani's spirits up. Martin went to Bamras every day.

"At the time, I thought I was going almost more for social reasons, to show him that we were paying attention and that we cared about him," he said. "Medically, he wasn't at risk."

Martin had written orders for chest X-rays to be shot every few days, to be sure Urbani's lungs were staying clear. The first few were fine. Then one, midway in the second week, was not. For the first time, he could see opaque infiltrates on the film.

Urbani's condition began to slide. Martin began listening to the daily teleconferences that linked the WHO and CDC teams working on SARS around the world, hoping for word of a treatment that might make a difference. He tried antibiotics to protect against the start of a secondary bacterial infection, newly developed antivirals, steroids because Hong Kong thought they were useful. Nothing helped. Urbani's oxygen levels were steadily declining. In the second week, they put him on a mask that forced air into his lungs.

"He would go for a day and be great, and then have a few bad days, and then a good day," Martin said. "He was strong, so strong. And mentally, he was always there."

Until, briefly, he wasn't. Pressurized oxygen is difficult to tolerate for long. The compressor noise is loud and intimate, and the whooshing air dries out the mouth and throat. For whatever reason, on a day when he had been in the hospital for more than two weeks, Urbani lifted off his oxygen mask, and his lungs collapsed.

Martin was not there. He arrived to find the Italian physician sedated and on a ventilator. The intubation had been smooth and quick, and his blood-oxygen levels were back to acceptable levels. But it was the beginning of an irreversible slide.

"He went two or three good days," Martin said. "And, you know, you're always grasping at straws. I remember thinking, in just a couple of days, he's going to turn the corner. We'll keep him comfortable, we'll do good medical care, and we'll just wait for him to come around."

He never did.

Dowell had returned to Bangkok. He and Martin were both experienced clinicians, but neither was a critical-care specialist. They had asked the WHO for extra help, and the agency had sent an Australian doctor whose specialty was intensive care. On the morning of March 29, she met with Martin to go over Urbani's condition. He had had a bad night, and she had had trouble keeping him oxygenated; she wanted Martin to know the details before she left for a few hours' break.

From the nursing station, Martin looked through the double set of windows. Urbani was lying peacefully, and there were nurses in the room with him. He picked up the phone to report to Dowell—and out of the corner of his eye, he saw one of the nurses spring toward Urbani's bed. Martin dropped the phone and ran, out of the nursing station, through the robing room for the second set of layers, and in with Urbani. The Italian's heart had stopped. They pounced on him with defibrillator paddles, and within a minute brought him back.

A cardiac arrest is never good news, but a minute is a short amount of time to be without oxygen; brain tissue starts to die after four minutes have passed. The more troubling thing was that Martin had no idea why Urbani had coded. Without knowing the reason for the heart attack, it was difficult to predict whether it would happen again.

He went back out to the nursing station, called Dowell, and began searching for Urbani's lab results from that morning, hoping to find some clue to the arrest in his blood chemistry. With his head in the chart, he heard one of the nurses bang on the window. He looked up. Urbani had coded again.

This time, getting him back took twenty minutes, an impossible length of time to be without a reliable heart rhythm. Still, Urbani rebounded: his pulse rate surged and stabilized, and his blood-oxygen began to creep back up. The team were uneasy, though, and so they stayed by his bedside. There was a moment's normalcy, and then his heart failed a third time.

Dowell had arrived at the hospital, but had no time to gown and glove. He grabbed a mask and slid into the walled nurses' station. Through the double windows, he could see Martin and a Bamras doctor and a succession of nurses, leaning stiff-armed over Urbani to give him chest compressions, backing away while one of them tried the defibrillator, waiting to see if the rhythm took hold, and then rushing in with compressions again.

The Thai doctor climbed on the bed for extra leverage. She was soaked with sweat, and her mask slipped. The sight jarred Martin out of his trance of urgency. He realized the risks the staff were running. He pulled her off the bed. She fought him. He pushed her out the door, and vaulted on the bed to take her place.

"Nobody wanted to lose Carlo," Martin said. "Nobody wanted to see him die."

After more than an hour, Martin and the nurses stepped back from the bed. There was no hint of a pulse. Urbani lay gray and unmoving. At 11:45 in the morning, they pronounced him dead.

———

Three days after Urbani died, the WHO's chief of communicable diseases announced that there had been no new cases of SARS in Vietnam for eight days. In mainland China, Hong Kong, and Canada, cases continued to climb, but it appeared the country that was the first to raise the alarm on the disease would be the first to beat it.

One day later—it was April 2—an older man named Bui Duc Khiem was carried by ambulance to Bach Mai Hospital from a town named Ninh Binh, ninety-five kilometers south of Hanoi. He was tired and achy, and had a high fever, and his chest X-ray showed lung infiltrates.

The investigators went to interview him. Vietnam's SARS outbreak had been so closely associated with the French Hospital that it was unsettling to hear of a possible case coming from so far away. What they discovered was dismaying. Bui did have a connection to the French Hospital outbreak: His daughter had had an appendectomy there in March, and he had visited her. But it also seemed possible that he had started an outbreak of his own: He had been sick with the symptoms of SARS, in his hometown, for at least ten days.

For half of that time, he had been in Ninh Binh Hospital, suffering from achiness and a high fever. Doctors there had attempted to transfer him to Bach Mai, which had been designated the SARS isolation center for the entire country, but the doctors at Bach Mai had turned him away, saying he did not have all the symptoms that marked a case. Dutifully, Bui had gone home. In Ninh Binh, he was a dignitary: Before he retired, he had been a highly placed official in the local People's Committee, holding a position equivalent to deputy mayor. Hearing that he had returned from Hanoi, still ill, relatives and friends had passed by the house to bring gifts and pay their respects. After three days, feeling worse than ever, he had returned to Ninh Binh Hospital. Doctors there had taken a second chest X-ray. Spotting the distinctive signs of inflammation, they sent him back to Hanoi and insisted that he be admitted. This time, the doctors at Bach Mai agreed.

Meanwhile, at Ninh Binh Hospital, Bui's doctor—a woman named Cuong, who was chief of internal medicine—had developed a fever and cough of her own. Fearing she had been infected, she put herself into isolation. Her staff and her husband, who was also a doctor, had all quarantined themselves in their homes.

The doctor's case was a clear indication that a second outbreak might be starting—and this one, unlike the French Hospital, had the potential to infect a wide community. The only people who had had contact with Johnny Chen, once he became infectious, were the doctors and nurses within one institution. But by Bui's estimate, more than a hundred people had passed through his house, and some of them had come from fifty kilometers away. The only way to find any new cases, and to keep them from spreading the disease, was to track them all down.

Joel and Dan headed south for Ninh Binh, along with Dr. Bach Huy Anh of the health ministry and Peter Horby, a British infectious disease physician who had been sent by WHO to augment Brudon's staff. The narrow road south was one lane in each direction, though "lane" was a discretionary concept to the overloaded trucks and motorbikes that leapfrogged each other down the center line and along the shoulders. It was spring, and the wet rice paddies that ran up to the road on both sides were filigreed with the incandescent green of new shoots. The villages lay back from the road, small clusters of narrow, four-story concrete houses painted sky-blue and lavender, next to walled cemeteries that held above-ground graves roofed in yellow and red. Forty kilometers out of Hanoi, the landscape changed suddenly: Narrow volcanic ridges, rough and sharp-edged, jutted out of the ground abruptly. One of them towered over the north end of Ninh Binh, topped by a Christian cross.

Ninh Binh Hospital lay in the south end of town, a two-story building that was shaped like a backwards E and fringed with fretwork balconies plastered a milky pink. The staff had prepared for the team's coming. They had washed down the rooms, using bleach as a disinfectant, and when Horby perched on the edge of a table the residue ate a hole in his trousers. The staff were also clearly unnerved to be meeting researchers from Hanoi, the center of the outbreak. They showed up wearing surgical masks—useless against viruses, but a reliable indicator of their fear.

On the drive down, the team had decided on a two-pronged approach. They needed to find Bui's contacts, to break the chain of transmission. But to ensure there would be no additional outbreaks, they needed to coach the hospital staff in infection-control protocols: who was at risk from patients, when they needed gowns and gloves, and what sort of masks to wear. They had brought boxes of N-95s, donated by *Médecins Sans frontières,* that had to be fitted to each wearer. They launched a training session on the spot. By the time the training session was over, half of the staff had sheepishly taken their masks off.

That night, the team negotiated a system of observation with the local communes, which were political committees that linked together households in a neighborhood. Volunteers would visit twice a day for

fourteen days to make sure none of Bui's hundred visitors were feverish or coughing, and would report them if they were. The most critical contacts, though, were Bui's family. The team wanted to do those
interviews themselves.

Bui lived a half-block off the road through the center of Ninh Binh,
in an ochre house that had a bicycle shop on the ground floor. The
next morning, the team set out to visit. The household was Bui's wife,
his son-in-law—the husband of the daughter who had been in the
French Hospital—and two teenaged nieces. The wife and the son-in-
law appeared fine, though Joel took their blood and swabbed their
throats to gather samples for the record. The two nieces were reluc-
tant to meet the investigators and had to be called down from an upstairs room. Their arrival downstairs showed why: They were feverish
and flushed. The team popped N-95 masks on them, and hustled
them into the van to get them into isolation at the hospital; they fitted
masks on the wife and son-in-law as well.

The next day, the son-in-law spiked a fever and joined the nieces in
the isolation ward. Three days afterward, one of the political volunteers came to the hospital asking for the Hanoi visitors. On his daily
rounds, he had found a friend of Bui's, a thirty-year-old man named
Luong who lived with his parents and brother in an alley twenty yards
from Bui's house. Luong drove a van for a living, and he had been in
Ho Chi Minh City for several days. But he had returned the previous
night, and he was not feeling well.

Luong was the first case turned up by the volunteer interrogators.
The team rushed to evaluate him. He was sweating and feverish, and
clearly unwell. They swabbed his throat and took his blood, fitted a
mask to his face, and sent him off to Ninh Binh Hospital on the back
of a motorbike.

———

Luong, who survived, was Vietnam's last recognized case of SARS.
Twenty days later, after two incubation periods had passed without
new cases, the WHO declared the country SARS-free. The place
where the epidemic had come to light became the first to fight it off.

Other countries followed suit. China, which had fueled the epidemic by denying its origins for five months, rallied in April under great international pressure. It placed tens of thousands of people under forced quarantine and deployed roving teams of health workers empowered to stop people on the street and test them for fever. At one point, using armed forces members working around the clock, it built a 1,000-bed quarantine hospital from an empty field, in a week. Its measures were so aggressive that, though it had more than half the cases in the epidemic, it had only three times as many as Hong Kong, in a population two hundred times Hong Kong's size. The United States, which received Urbani's early warning—and to the CDC's knowledge was never visited by a highly infectious patient such as Johnny Chen—was equally fortunate: It had, in the end, only twenty-nine cases of SARS.

Other areas were not so lucky. Canada, where Kwan Sui Chu brought the disease February 23, battled repeated outbreaks, almost all of them in hospitals. Two Toronto hospitals were shut by Ontario's public health authority, while visitors were barred from all others—and from nursing homes, prisons, and long-term care facilities—unless they were relatives of sick children or critically ill adults. All hospital doors were locked and guarded, and all hospital employees were required to wear gloves, gowns, masks, and protective eyewear for the entire time they were at work.

Nevertheless, the disease continued to leak out. In mid-April, more than thirty cases were discovered among members of a Toronto charismatic religious group, the Bukas-Loob Sa Diyos community. One of its members, an eighty-two-year-old man, had been treated in the emergency department of Scarborough Grace Hospital; he sat near a seventy-six-year-old man who had shared a room with Kwan's son, Tse. Tse died March 13, and the seventy-six-year-old on March 21. The eighty-two-year-old died April 1, and when his friends and family mingled at his wake and funeral, SARS spread among them. They unknowingly passed the disease to an American man who attended a retreat with the group and fell ill after returning home to Pennsylvania. In late May, SARS flared again in Toronto, starting with a ninety-nine-year-old man who was brought to North York

General Hospital north of the city with a broken pelvis. When he developed pneumonia after being hospitalized, it was not recognized as SARS. The outbreak that began with him spread to seventy-eight other patients and health care workers before being shut down. And in June, twenty women and their newborn children were quarantined after a medical student who helped deliver the babies came down with SARS two days after being released from a ten-day quarantine.

Taiwan, which appeared at first to escape the epidemic, fared worse. From late February to April, the island had only two dozen cases of the disease, all carried over the straits by business travelers from the Chinese mainland. They were all found quickly and treated, though one of them passed the infection to a nurse and three family members. And then the outbreak seemed to stop. It is possible the disease simmered without being noticed. It is probable that a false sense of confidence over vanquishing it—combined with a lesser degree of foreign help at first, because Taiwan, in a bow to China, is not recognized by the WHO—led to a relaxation of vigilance.

On April 16, a forty-two-year-old man who ran the laundry at Taipei's Municipal Ho Ping Hospital was admitted to a ward in his own institution with a fever and diarrhea. The man, who died April 29, lived in a room in the hospital basement and spent his free time in the emergency department, where some of his friends worked. By the time authorities realized he was a SARS case, the disease had seeded itself throughout the hospital; staff, patients, and visitors had all been exposed. More than three hundred additional cases followed, in eight other hospitals and in the community as well. Taiwan's health minister stepped down, and several hundred nurses and other health workers resigned from their jobs rather than risk treating SARS patients.

The last case in the cluster developed symptoms on June 15. It was the last case of SARS in Taiwan, and it proved to be the last in the epidemic as well. On July 5, WHO director-general Brundtland declared the fight over, for the time being.

"We do not mark the end of SARS today, but we observe a milestone: The global SARS outbreak has been contained," she said in Geneva, adding: "This is not the time to relax our vigilance. The world must remain on high alert."

Between November 2002 and July 2003, there were 8,098 cases of SARS worldwide, and 774 deaths. Twenty-one percent of the victims were health care workers.

In Vietnam, there were sixty-three cases, more than half of them doctors and nurses, and five deaths. But there were anomalies also. Though more than a third of the victims had been hospitalized at Bach Mai, SARS never spread to the staff there. Nor, after the six initial cases, did it spread in Ninh Binh, despite the prolonged face-to-face contact between Mr. Bui and his doctor and at least one hundred others. At some point, for some inexplicable reason, SARS had simply stopped.

"We can't understand why it didn't spread throughout Vietnam," Joel said. "Granted, the Vietnamese government did a remarkable job containing it, and the team did too. But I don't know who the credit should be given to, for ending the outbreak. Was it really what we did? Was there something in the population? Vietnam is an enigma."

July–September
2003

THE FIRST TROPICAL STORM OF 2003 hit Atlanta on July 1. By early afternoon, the sky was the color of asphalt. The rain fell with force, straight down, as opaque as fiberglass, turning the ramps of parking decks into waterfalls. In the lobby of an office building on the northeast side of the city, men and women in uniform arrived dripping, huddling under umbrellas and shaking the water off their shiny military shoes.

July 1 was not a Wednesday, the CDC's mandatory-uniform day. The Commissioned Corps officers fighting their way through the weather were dressed for a special occasion: They were being promoted. Eighty-eight corps members, including members of the 2002 EIS class, had passed competitive requirements to move up a grade.

Kirsten Ernst, the nurse with the double master's degrees who had led one of the West Nile investigations—and who belonged to the group who had no objections to wearing the uniform—had organized a promotion ceremony with Danice Eaton, a classmate who was a behavioral science Ph.D. It began with a color guard, and a choir of corps members singing the words to the Public Health Service anthem ("The mission of our service / Is known the world around . . ."). The guest of honor, there to shake hands and button on the shoulder boards indicating the new ranks, was an HHS regional administrator and PHS rear admiral named J. Jarrett Clinton.

Clinton was a tall, slender man with straight posture and a cool, correct manner. His congratulatory speech was polite rather than rousing; he praised the officers being promoted but lamented that their service was so little known.

"We hide under our own basket by not talking about the Commissioned Corps," he said. "The song says we are known around the world, but you and I know that we are not. We can walk among lay people in uniform and they will ask, 'Which ship are you on?' "

Fourteen of the 2002 class had waded through the rain for the ceremony. More than that had been promoted, but they were not all free to come. Claire Newbern was in Philadelphia; Nolan Lee was in Los Angeles, tracking the still-expanding epidemic of drug-resistant staph. Some of the Atlanta officers had been dragooned into the EOC, including Jennifer Gordon Wright, who had planned to come to the ceremony until she was abruptly assigned down to the bunker. SARS was fading, but another illness had taken its place in the headlines: monkeypox, a disease related to smallpox that had never appeared in the Western Hemisphere before. Seventy-one people in six states were sick, and thirty had been given smallpox vaccinations to protect them. The war room staff were tracing the shipment of exotic pets that had brought monkeypox into the country. Joel Montgomery was tracking the new disease in the field.

Sami Gottlieb and Scott Filler were not at the ceremony either. Sami was at home, and Scott was rushing through work in Chamblee so he could join her. Twelve days earlier, she had given birth to their daughter, Maia.

The ceremony was being held off-campus, in one of the twenty-some satellite locations the CDC rented around Atlanta. The setting, a plain gray conference room cut in half by a folding wall and furnished with a wood-veneer podium and snap-together chairs, was unexpectedly moving: It suggested how anonymous the disease detective corps remained.

Or perhaps how interchangeable. Such ceremonies were usually held in Auditorium B, the big modern conference room at headquarters. Auditorium B was booked, though. Inside it, at the same time the class of 2002 were being promoted, the seventy-eight members of the EIS class of 2003 were starting their summer training course.

———

The EIS has no formal graduation ceremony: There is no equivalent of moving a mortarboard tassel from one side to the other, or exchanging a short white lab coat for a long one. Every July, the officers ending their two-year term in the group quietly move over to whatever full-time jobs they have found at the CDC or elsewhere. Equally without fanfare, the first-years become second-years, ready to start serving as mentors once the entering first-years finish their month-long summer training.

The closest thing to a rite of passage is the annual EIS Conference, the four-day gathering in April that has not changed substantially since Alex Langmuir staged the first one in 1952. It is a fast-moving scientific meeting, a single session held in a large ballroom with a different speaker every twenty minutes; each gets ten minutes to present a paper and ten more to answer questions from the audience. The presenters are always current EIS officers. The program is constantly at risk of being overloaded by second-years because it represents one of their last opportunities to present a scientific paper at a major meeting, a mark they are supposed to hit before their EIS stint ends. But in April 2003, fifty of the ninety-eight papers came from the 2002 class, along with twenty-two of the thirty posters—a less prestigious form of presentation in which authors mount their papers on boards and stand nearby to discuss them with passersby. The first session of the conference was conducted by CDC director Julie Gerberding. For the first paper in the first session, the organizers chose Martha Iwamoto's investigation into organ transplants and West Nile.

EIS officers were expected to attend the conference to the degree their jobs allowed, and their supervisors were supposed to relax schedules for the week to let them come if possible. The rules would have worked, except that this April, SARS was still in full roar. Instead, the group grabbed breaks from their EOC stints to make their own presentations and listen to their friends' papers. When they could, they sat in the audience, along with hundreds of EIS alumni who had returned for the week.

Almost nine hundred alumni still worked at the CDC, so it was easy for them to come to the meeting. Others had made careers in state health departments, academic medicine, public health school faculties, and hospital staffs. They had spread out to forty-nine states (none, mysteriously, in Arkansas); Washington, D.C., Puerto Rico, and the U.S. Virgin Islands; and forty countries, with a substantial contingent in Geneva at the WHO. When they came back to attend the conference, they demonstrated in a quite literal way how far EIS officers would go to support each other.

"There's a tremendous esprit de corps that builds up," said Ralph Henderson, a physician who joined the EIS in 1965, worked in Africa, and then was loaned to the WHO for most of his career. He had returned to Atlanta in retirement, where he was designing an EIS-like program for the WHO. Whenever he was in town, he attended the Tuesday morning seminars, always introducing himself as a "retired EIS officer."

It had been easy to see, over their first year of service, what being at the CDC did for the EIS members: It gave them concentrated training and a credential that would launch the next phase of their careers. The assembled alumni were a glimpse of what, in turn, the EIS did for the CDC. While they were there, they provided a reliable supply of fresh frontline workers—even if the work they were assigned sometimes made them feel more like grunts than like the Green Berets they were supposed to resemble. Mentoring them forced their supervisors, and the whole agency, to stay flexible enough to anticipate the unpredictable twists of investigations. They graduated, if they left the CDC, into an ad hoc network that stayed engaged with the agency, understood how it operated, and was almost uniformly loyal to it.

"These people are in touch; they're all out there networking with each other," Henderson went on. "The institution becomes far more effective because it's got hands and eyes everywhere."

———

Its energetic response to the SARS epidemic had thrown a glow of good reputation over the CDC. To the longtime staff, the positive regard felt like a pleasant vindication after the battering the agency took over anthrax. Canada and the European Union had both announced plans to establish disease-control agencies of their own in imitation of the CDC. The WHO's incoming director-general, Dr. Lee Jong-Wook, had endorsed Henderson's plan to launch a training program for young professionals from developing countries, a move that would give the organization its own disease-detective corps.

So it seemed ironic that, while the CDC was being acclaimed abroad, parts of it were being altered at home. Two days after the promotion ceremony, HHS Secretary Thompson and Surgeon General Carmona announced plans to "transform" the six-thousand-member Commissioned Corps. Some of the changes, enhancing scholarships and recruiting, were benign. Others promised to have a direct impact on the EIS class and the other corps members at the CDC.

There would be new emphasis on more frequent wearing of the uniform, which in a break with tradition would include fatigues for the first time. There would be physical fitness requirements; after 2004, corps members who could not meet exertion and body-fat standards would lose their chance at promotion. Every corps member, no matter how senior, would become subject to immediate emergency deployment just as EIS officers were. There were changes to the health insurance and the promotion system, and rumors of mandatory transfers away from the CDC into other HHS agencies. The overall effect, from the HHS side, was to create a group that was more like the military, in philosophy and organization at least if not in mission: lean, mobile, and versatile, owing allegiance not to the individual HHS agencies but to the corps itself. From the point of view of the EIS class, who joined the corps primarily because it was the price of admission to the CDC, the changes were disturbing. They felt as though the ground were shifting under their feet.

In the midst of the unforeseen changes, the group was thankful that one forecast event had not come to pass: Throughout their year of service, there had been no hint of bioterrorism. There had been no repeat of the anthrax attacks, and no biological weapons were deployed against the coalition forces fighting in Iraq. The debate over whether Iraq had possessed such weapons would grow steadily more bitter.

As the proximate risk of attack appeared to fade, demands for immediate protection did as well. The national smallpox vaccination campaign, which had expected to inoculate up to 450,000 health care workers and first responders, by July enrolled fewer than 37,000 volunteers. Since the announcement of its launch in December, the program had grown steadily more controversial. The Institute of Medicine—an arm of the National Academy of Sciences, which advises Congress on health policy—twice called on the CDC to pause and reevaluate the program. At the same time, new risks of vaccination emerged. Several young military members experienced mild heart inflammation after getting the vaccine; several older health workers had heart attacks afterward, and three died. The inflammation cases were mild, and the heart attacks were believed to have been complicated by diabetes, obesity, and other signs of poor health in the older recipients. Still, cardiac events after smallpox vaccination had never been observed before—largely because, when the vaccine was last broadly used, it had mostly been given to toddlers—and the news put a further brake on the vaccination campaign. Across the country, health workers whom planners had expected to demand the vaccine instead backed away from it, frightened off by the imbalance between its known risk of side effects and its uncertain benefit of protection against an attack that might not come.

A few of the volunteers were in the EIS class. In the winter, they had been asked whether they would take the shot, if the opportunity were offered. In early spring, the opportunity came. Kirsten and several other officers stepped up.

"Right away I started with the aches and the soreness and the night sweat and the fevers, but that was all expected," Kirsten said. "Then about day eight or day nine, my entire shoulder swelled up. I couldn't lower my arm because my lymph nodes were so swollen. But the vaccination program said it was within normal bounds for reactions. And two days later, I was fine."

Jennifer had considered taking the vaccine but rejected it. Her infant daughter had eczema, which was a known contraindication to smallpox vaccination; the disease paved the way for uncontrolled vaccine reactions because it disrupted the immune response in the skin. If she passed the vaccine virus on to her child, she risked giving the baby a potentially fatal infection. Evaluating whether to take the vaccine had led her to think back to the bioterrorism training in their first EIS weeks, and to consider what the true shape of their risks might be.

"I worry more about what is already out there than what people conjure up in a lab," she said. "I worry about SARS, and about influenza mutating and causing another 1918-type of epidemic. We were lucky that monkeypox wasn't something like Ebola that is more deadly and more transmissible person to person. And if something like that happened, we are still the first who would be sent out."

———

The end of their first year introduced another destabilizing element into the lives of the 2002 class: the acute awareness that, before another twelve months elapsed, they would need to find jobs.

EIS service was considered the surest path into a career at the CDC, but there was no guarantee of employment at its end. Uncertainty over whether they would be offered jobs would begin haunting officers early in their second year, and end only when their supervisors invited them to stay or confessed that there was no extra room in the budget. The brinksmanship bore particularly hard on the EIS members who were Ph.D.s. For research scientists, the natural alternative to a job at the CDC was a university faculty position—but each year, the academic hiring season ended long before CDC supervisors learned whether they would have jobs available. The fallback position was for an EIS member to take a position elsewhere in the agency, a maneuver that effectively asked a scientist to value CDC employment over his or her own expertise. In late summer 2003, Joel began to wonder whether he was facing that choice.

"I'd like to stay with Special Pathogens," he said one morning. Monkeypox was over; he was taking a break from co-authoring a paper on SARS in Vietnam. "I enjoy the work I'm doing, and I've got projects that are all kind of beginning now. It would be nice to see some of them to completion."

The difficult reality, only now becoming clear, was that the projects they found most absorbing would not end when the group's EIS term did. If they found permanent jobs in the offices where they were already working, they were likely to see their work through to publication in a scientific journal, an event that would count heavily on their resumes. If they were forced to find work elsewhere—in the CDC, or outside it—they might end their service by turning their work and their chance of publication over to someone else. If before they moved they had already started to write a scientific paper, their supervisors might allow them to take it away and finish it, even though the research results technically belonged not to them personally but to the office they were exiting. Taking the paper with them, though, would mean writing up results and wrestling with co-authors in late nights and weekends as they struggled to learn new jobs.

Scott was in that position. An underlying assumption of his malaria-in-pregnancy study had proved inaccurate: The rate of HIV infection in the area was not as high as the CDC malaria branch had supposed. How long the study lasted was determined by how rapidly HIV-positive mothers enrolled in it; the longer it took to find them, the more time would pass before the study ended. The project had been designed to last two years; now it seemed likely to stretch for three, going well into 2005. But in summer 2004, Scott would have to find a permanent job—in malaria if the branch had an opening, or somewhere else if not.

"EIS has been everything I wanted it to be," he said. "My expectations were for getting international health experience, and learning how to run studies overseas, and that's most of what I have done. But a lot of how I will feel about this, when it is over, will depend on how the job situation works out. If I stay at the branch and I can get the study done and then move on to work on other things, then my experience will have been absolutely perfect."

The enthusiasm the EIS class felt for continuing their work at the CDC was poignant, because they would graduate into a harsh professional environment. The researchers who had been lured into public health by the challenge of eradicating smallpox were approaching the end of their civil service careers. Almost half of the CDC's doctors and biological-science researchers would qualify for retirement in 2008. It was unclear how many would be replaced. The anthrax attacks, and the boost in federal funding they had brought, had created a boom market in public health jobs. The CDC and state health departments were competing against expanding university faculties and new consulting firms for the small pool of public-health graduates, and losing. There were only half as many employees under forty at the CDC as there were employees over forty. The stress on the remaining public health workers was intense. For the 2002 class, the forecast of a more difficult future made the remaining days of their EIS service more precious.

"I got a lot of experience in things I hadn't done before, things that I was eager to learn," Sami said. It was late summer. Maia was growing into an enchanting baby, with Sami's wide blue eyes and a fringe of Scott's dark hair. Sami was battling the fatigue of being a new parent to prepare a talk on listeriosis for a national scientific meeting. She would fly to New Orleans to present it while still on maternity leave.

"But the biggest thing about EIS is not even what you learn," she added. "It's the community it places you in. You call people up, and you say you're an EIS officer, and they welcome you into this intellectual family. You pass through these challenges, and you become part of the network, and it makes your job so much easier to do."

———

Outside the promotion ceremony, Tropical Storm Bill was still bucketing down. Inside, Rear Admiral Clinton was building up to the finish of his remarks, the last thing he would say to the 2002 EIS officers before he delivered the insignia and handshakes that would formalize their move into their second year.

He gestured to the gold banner hanging behind him, next to the U.S. flag. It bore the 205-year-old symbol of the Public Health Service: a caduceus, the millennia-old sign of the healing professions, crossed over an anchor wound about with a heavy chain.

"How many of you have a boat?" he asked. "Well, then, I think you will understand this. When you drop an anchor, it is very important to have the line straight so the anchor digs in well. One of the things we always fear is that the line gets hooked around the fluke of the anchor; then, if there is any tension on the line, the anchor won't hold. That is referred to as a fouled anchor. That is what's on this flag.

"Now, a fouled anchor is a symbol," he said. "It means that a boat is in trouble. So our symbol is the caduceus, the ancient symbol of medicine, combined with the symbol for trouble. At the intersection where those two meet, that is where our work happens. That is our job."

NOTES ON SOURCES AND SELECTED BIBLIOGRAPHY

This book is based on 195 interviews with 133 present and former staff of the U.S. Centers for Disease Control and Prevention, longtime observers of the agency, scientific collaborators of its staff, and others. The interviewees included 94 members of the Epidemic Intelligence Service, past and present, in the United States and in other countries. I am deeply indebted to all of them.

I conducted all the interviews on which this book is based. The majority were conducted face-to-face, taped, and then transcribed, usually by professional transcriptionists but occasionally by myself. Some interviews were conducted in person and recorded by hand in notebooks, but not taped, and a few were conducted by phone. Many subjects agreed to be interviewed several times; the record is seven. I appreciate the access they offered and the patience and good humor they exhibited in the face of my persistent questions.

Direct quotations were taken only from interview transcripts or notes. The only exception to this is quotations from Alex Langmuir and the lone quote by Joseph Mountin; these are drawn from Langmuir's published writings. Descriptions of EIS members' thoughts or feelings are paraphrased from their own characterizations. Reconstructions of events that I did not witness are based on the memories of two or more participants. Their accounts of EIS investigations were checked against scientific papers written by EIS members and published in medical and public health journals; contemporaneous accounts in local, national, and foreign newspapers and newsmagazines; CDC archival materials and other government records; and the personal papers, diaries, and photographs of EIS graduates.

My understanding of the diseases and other health problems encountered by EIS members, and of the milieux in which they worked, was informed by the following books, reports, and scientific articles. I am grateful to all the authors for their scholarship.

SELECTED BIBLIOGRAPHY

Kaposi's sarcoma and Pneumocystis pneumonia among homosexual men—New York City and California. 1981. *MMWR Morb Mortal Wkly Rep* 30 (25):305–8.

Pneumocystis pneumonia—Los Angeles. 1981. *MMWR Morb Mortal Wkly Rep* 30 (21):250–2.

A cluster of Kaposi's sarcoma and Pneumocystis carinii pneumonia among homosexual male residents of Los Angeles and Orange Counties, California. 1982. *MMWR Morb Mortal Wkly Rep* 31 (23):305–7.

Toxic epidemic syndrome, Spain, 1981. Toxic Epidemic Syndrome Study Group. 1982. *Lancet* 2 (8300):697–702.

Update on Kaposi's sarcoma and opportunistic infections in previously healthy persons—United States. 1982. *MMWR Morb Mortal Wkly Rep* 31 (22):294, 300–1.

Toxic oil syndrome. 1983. *Lancet* 1 (8336):1257–8.

Transmission of multidrug-resistant tuberculosis among immuno-compromised persons in a correctional system—New York, 1991. 1992. *MMWR Morb Mortal Wkly Rep* 41 (28):507–509.

Joint Emergency Winter Humanitarian Needs Assessment Mission to Northern Iraq, October 9–16, 1992. 1992. Washington, DC: Office of U.S. Foreign Disaster Assistance, U.S. Agency for International Development.

Public health impact of Rwandan refugee crisis: what happened in Goma, Zaire, in July, 1994? Goma Epidemiology Group. 1995. *Lancet* 345 (8946):339–44.

Historical Perspectives: History of CDC. 1996. *MMWR Morb Mortal Wkly Rep* 45 (25):526–30.

Four pediatric deaths from community-acquired methicillin-resistant staphylococcus aureus—Minnesota and North Dakota, 1997–1999. 1999. *MMWR Morb Mortal Wkly Rep* 48 (32):707–10.

HIV-related tuberculosis in a transgender network—Baltimore,

Maryland, and New York City area, 1998–2000. 2000. *MMWR Morb Mortal Wkly Rep* 49 (15):317–20.

Cluster of tuberculosis cases among exotic dancers and their close contacts—Kansas, 1994–2000. 2001. *MMWR Morb Mortal Wkly Rep* 50 (15):291–3.

Methicillin-resistant Staphylococcus aureus skin or soft tissue infections in a state prison—Mississippi, 2000. 2001. *MMWR Morb Mortal Wkly Rep* 50 (42):919–22.

Chagas disease after organ transplantation—United States, 2001. 2002. *MMWR Morb Mortal Wkly Rep* 51 (10):210–2.

Considerations for Viral Disease Education: Lessons Learned and Future Strategies. 2002. Washington, DC: National Academy of Sciences.

Investigation of blood transfusion recipients with West Nile virus infections. 2002. *MMWR Morb Mortal Wkly Rep* 51 (36):823.

Investigations of West Nile virus infections in recipients of blood transfusions. 2002. *MMWR Morb Mortal Wkly Rep* 51 (43):973–4.

Outbreak of listeriosis—northeastern United States, 2002. 2002. *MMWR Morb Mortal Wkly Rep* 51 (42):950–1.

Update: Investigations of West Nile virus infections in recipients of organ transplantation and blood transfusion. 2002. *MMWR Morb Mortal Wkly Rep* 51 (37):833–6.

Update: Investigations of West Nile virus infections in recipients of organ transplantation and blood transfusion—Michigan, 2002. 2002. *MMWR Morb Mortal Wkly Rep* 51 (39):879.

West Nile virus infection in organ donor and transplant recipients—Georgia and Florida, 2002. 2002. *MMWR Morb Mortal Wkly Rep* 51 (35):790.

Cardiac deaths after a mass smallpox vaccination campaign—New York City, 1947. 2003. *MMWR Morb Mortal Wkly Rep* 52 (39):933–6.

Cluster of severe acute respiratory syndrome cases among protected health-care workers—Toronto, Canada, April 2003. 2003. *MMWR Morb Mortal Wkly Rep* 52 (19):433–6.

COA Position Statement on DHHS Transformation Plan for the PHS Commissioned Corps. 2003. Washington, DC: Commissioned Officers Association of the U.S. Public Health Service.

Detection of West Nile virus in blood donations—United States, 2003. 2003. *MMWR Morb Mortal Wkly Rep* 52 (32):769–72.

Homeland Insecurity: Building the expertise to defend America from bioterrorism. 2003. Washington, DC: Partnership for Public Service.

Manual circular—Commissioned Corps personnel, PHS No. 375. 2003. Division of Commissioned Personnel, Department of Health and Human Services.

Methicillin-resistant Staphylococcus aureus infections among competitive sports participants—Colorado, Indiana, Pennsylvania, and Los Angeles County, 2000–2003. 2003. *MMWR Morb Mortal Wkly Rep* 52 (33):793–5.

Methicillin-resistant Staphylococcus aureus infections in correctional facilities—Georgia, California, and Texas, 2001–2003. 2003. *MMWR Morb Mortal Wkly Rep* 52 (41):992–6.

Outbreak of severe acute respiratory syndrome—worldwide, 2003. 2003. *MMWR Morb Mortal Wkly Rep* 52 (11):226–8.

Outbreaks of community-associated methicillin-resistant Staphylococcus aureus skin infections—Los Angeles County, California, 2002–2003. 2003. *MMWR Morb Mortal Wkly Rep* 52 (5):88.

Revised U.S. surveillance case definition for severe acute respiratory syndrome (SARS) and update on SARS cases—United States and worldwide, December 2003. 2003. *MMWR Morb Mortal Wkly Rep* 52 (49):1202–6.

U.S. Congress House of Representatives. 2003. Committee on Government Reform. *Serving the Underserved in the 21st Century: The Need for a Stronger, More Responsive Public Health Service Commissioned Corps.* October 30, 2003.

Severe acute respiratory syndrome—Singapore, 2003. 2003. *MMWR Morb Mortal Wkly Rep* 52 (18):405–11.

Severe acute respiratory syndrome—Taiwan, 2003. 2003. *MMWR Morb Mortal Wkly Rep* 52 (20):461–6.

Surveillance for acute insecticide-related illness associated with mosquito-control efforts—nine states, 1999–2002. 2003. *MMWR Morb Mortal Wkly Rep* 52 (27):629–34.

Transmission of hepatitis B and C viruses in outpatient settings—New York, Oklahoma, and Nebraska, 2000–2002. 2003. *MMWR Morb Mortal Wkly Rep* 52 (38):901–6.

Update: Detection of West Nile virus in blood donations—United States, 2003. 2003. *MMWR Morb Mortal Wkly Rep* 52 (38):916–9.

Update: Multistate outbreak of monkeypox—Illinois, Indiana, Kansas, Missouri, Ohio, and Wisconsin, 2003. 2003. *MMWR Morb Mortal Wkly Rep* 52 (27):642–6.

Update: Outbreak of severe acute respiratory syndrome—worldwide, 2003. 2003. *MMWR Morb Mortal Wkly Rep* 52 (12):241–6, 248.

Update: Outbreak of severe acute respiratory syndrome—worldwide, 2003. 2003. *MMWR Morb Mortal Wkly Rep* 52 (13):269–72.

Update: Severe acute respiratory syndrome—Toronto, Canada, 2003. 2003. *MMWR Morb Mortal Wkly Rep* 52 (23):547–50.

Update: Severe acute respiratory syndrome—United States, 2003. 2003. *MMWR Morb Mortal Wkly Rep* 52 (16):357–60.

Update: Severe acute respiratory syndrome—United States, May 28, 2003. 2003. *MMWR Morb Mortal Wkly Rep* 52 (21):500–1.

American Public Health Association. 1995. *Control of communicable diseases manual.* Washington, DC: American Public Health Association.

Baggett, H. C., T. W. Hennessy, R. Leman, C. Hamlin, D. Bruden, A. Reasonover, P. Martinez, and J. C. Butler. 2003. An outbreak of community-onset methicillin-resistant Staphylococcus aureus skin infections in southwestern Alaska. *Infect Control Hosp Epidemiol* 24 (6):397–402.

Biggerstaff, B. J., and L. R. Petersen. 2002. Estimated risk of West Nile virus transmission through blood transfusion during an epidemic in Queens, New York City. *Transfusion* 42 (8):1019–26.

Blendon, R. J., C. M. DesRoches, J. M. Benson, M. J. Herrmann, K. Taylor-Clark, and K. J. Weldon. 2003. The public and the smallpox threat. *N Engl J Med* 348 (5):426–32.

Bozzette, S. A., R. Boer, V. Bhatnagar, J. L. Brower, E. B. Keeler, S. C. Morton, and M. A. Stoto. 2003. A model for a smallpox-vaccination policy. *N Engl J Med* 348 (5):416–25.

Brachman, P. S. 1996. Alexander Duncan Langmuir. *Am J Epidemiol* 144 (8 Suppl):S74–5.

Breiman, R. F., M. R. Evans, W. Preiser, J. Maguire, A. Schnur, A. Li, H. Bekedam, and J. S. MacKenzie. 2003. Role of China in the quest to define and control severe acute respiratory syndrome. *Emerg Infect Dis* 9 (9):1037–41.

Buffington, J. 1999. Nonmedical doctoral-level scientists in the Centers for Disease Control and Prevention's Epidemic Intelligence Service, 1964–1997. *Am J Prev Med* 16 (4):341–345.

Burkholder, B. T., and M. J. Toole. 1995. Evolution of complex disasters. *Lancet* 346 (8981):1012–5.

Chen, R. T., and J. M. Lane. 2003. Myocarditis: the unexpected return of smallpox vaccine adverse events. *Lancet* 362 (9393):1345–6.

Das, D., D. Weiss, F. Mostashari, T. Treadwell, J. McQuiston, L. Hutwagner, A. Karpati, K. Bornschlegel, M. Seeman, R. Turcios, P. Terebuh, R. Curtis, R. Heffernan, and S. Balter. 2003. Enhanced drop-in syndromic surveillance in New York City following September 11, 2001. *J Urban Health* 80 (2 Suppl 1):i76–88.

Defoe, Daniel, and Louis A. Landa. 1990. *A journal of the plague year: being observations or memorials of the most remarkable occurrences, as well publick as private, which happened in London during the last Great Visitation in 1665*. The World's classics. Oxford and New York: Oxford University Press.

Des Forges, Alison Liebhafsky, Human Rights Watch, and Fédération internationale des droits de l'homme. 1999. *"Leave none to tell the story": genocide in Rwanda*. New York and Paris: Human Rights Watch; International Federation of Human Rights.

Desowitz, Robert S. 1991. *The malaria capers: more tales of parasites and people, research and reality*. New York: W. W. Norton.

Dewan, P. K., A. M. Fry, K. Laserson, B. C. Tierney, C. P. Quinn, J. A. Hayslett, L. N. Broyles, A. Shane, K. L. Winthrop, I. Walks, L. Siegel, T. Hales, V. A. Semenova, S. Romero-Steiner, C. Elie, R. Khabbaz, A. S. Khan, R. A. Hajjeh, and A. Schuchat. 2002. Inhalational anthrax outbreak among postal workers, Washington, D.C., 2001. *Emerg Infect Dis* 8 (10):1066–72.

Diamond, Jared M. 1997. *Guns, germs, and steel: the fates of human societies*. 1st ed. New York: W. W. Norton.

Dowell, S. F., A. Toko, C. Sita, R. Piarroux, A. Duerr, and B. A. Woodruff. 1995. Health and nutrition in centers for unaccompanied refugee children: experience from the 1994 Rwandan refugee crisis. *JAMA* 273 (22):1802–6.

Drexler, Madeline. 2002. *Secret agents: the menace of emerging infections*. Washington, DC: Joseph Henry Press.

Drosten, C., S. Gunther, W. Preiser, S. van der Werf, H. R. Brodt, S. Becker, H. Rabenau, M. Panning, L. Kolesnikova, R. A. Fouchier, A. Berger, A. M. Burguiere, J. Cinatl, M. Eickmann, N. Escriou, K. Grywna, S. Kramme, J. C. Manuguerra, S. Muller, V. Rickerts, M. Sturmer, S. Vieth, H. D. Klenk, A. D. Osterhaus, H. Schmitz, and H. W. Doerr. 2003. Identification of a novel coronavirus in patients with severe acute respiratory syndrome. *N Engl J Med* 348 (20):1967–76.

Dull, P. M., K. E. Wilson, B. Kournikakis, E. A. Whitney, C. A. Boulet, J. Y. Ho, J. Ogston, M. R. Spence, M. M. McKenzie, M. A. Phelan, T. Popovic, and D. Ashford. 2002. Bacillus anthracis aerosolization associated with a contaminated mail sorting machine. *Emerg Infect Dis* 8 (10):1044–7.

Eickhoff, T. C. 1996. Airborne disease: including chemical and biological warfare. *Am J Epidemiol* 144 (8 Suppl):S39–46.

Etheridge, Elizabeth W. 1992. *Sentinel for health: a history of the Centers for Disease Control*. Berkeley: University of California Press.

Fenner, Frank, and World Health Organization. 1988. *Smallpox and its eradication: History of international public health no. 6*. Geneva: World Health Organization.

Foege, W. H. 1996. Alexander D. Langmuir—his impact on public health. *Am J Epidemiol* 144 (8 Suppl):S11–5.

———. 2001. The wonder that is global health. *Nat Med* 7 (10):1095–6.

Foster, E. M. 1997. Historical overview of key issues in food safety. *Emerg Infect Dis* 3 (4):481–2.

Foster, S. O., and E. Gangarosa. 1996. Passing the epidemiologic torch from Farr to the world: the legacy of Alexander D. Langmuir. *Am J Epidemiol* 144 (8 Suppl):S65–73.

Francis, T., Jr., R. F. Korns, R. B. Voight, M. Boisen, F. M. Hemphill, J. A. Napier, and E. Tolchinsky. 1955. An evaluation of the

1954 poliomyelitis vaccine trials. *Am J Public Health* 45 (5, Part 2):1–63.

Fulginiti, V. A., A. Papier, J. M. Lane, J. M. Neff, and D. A. Henderson. 2003. Smallpox vaccination: a review, part I. Background, vaccination technique, normal vaccination and revaccination, and expected normal reactions. *Clin Infect Dis* 37 (2):241–50.

———. 2003. Smallpox vaccination: a review, part II. Adverse events. *Clin Infect Dis* 37 (2):251–71.

Garrett, Laurie. 1994. *The coming plague: newly emerging diseases in a world out of balance.* New York: Farrar, Straus and Giroux.

Gerberding, J. L. 2003. Faster . . . but fast enough? Responding to the epidemic of severe acute respiratory syndrome. *N Engl J Med* 348 (20):2030–1.

Giesecke, Johan. 2002. *Modern infectious disease epidemiology.* 2nd ed. London and New York: Arnold.

Goodman, R. A., C. F. Bauman, M. B. Gregg, J. F. Videtto, D. F. Stroup, and N. P. Chalmers. 1990. Epidemiologic field investigations by the Centers for Disease Control and Epidemic Intelligence Service, 1946–87. *Public Health Rep* 105 (6):604–10.

Gordis, Leon. 1996. *Epidemiology.* Philadelphia: W. B. Saunders.

Gottlieb, M. S. 2001. AIDS—past and future. *N Engl J Med* 344 (23):1788–91.

Gottlieb, M. S., R. Schroff, H. M. Schanker, J. D. Weisman, P. T. Fan, R. A. Wolf, and A. Saxon. 1981. Pneumocystis carinii pneumonia and mucosal candidiasis in previously healthy homosexual men: evidence of a new acquired cellular immunodeficiency. *N Engl J Med* 305 (24):1425–31.

Gourevitch, Philip. 1998. *We wish to inform you that tomorrow we will be killed with our families: stories from Rwanda.* New York: Farrar, Straus, and Giroux.

Greenberg, M. R. 2003. Public health, law, and local control: destruction of the US chemical weapons stockpile. *Am J Public Health* 93 (8):1222–6.

Gross-Schulman, S., D. Dassey, L. Mascola, and C. Anaya. 1998. Community-acquired methicillin-resistant Staphylococcus aureus. *JAMA* 280 (5):421–2.

Guarner, J., J. A. Jernigan, W. J. Shieh, K. Tatti, L. M. Flannagan, D. S. Stephens, T. Popovic, D. A. Ashford, B. A. Perkins, and S.

R. Zaki. 2003. Pathology and pathogenesis of bioterrorism-related inhalational anthrax. *Am J Pathol* 163 (2):701–9.

Harrington, T., M. J. Kuehnert, H. Kamel, R. S. Lanciotti, S. Hand, M. Currier, M. E. Chamberland, L. R. Petersen, and A. A. Marfin. 2003. West Nile virus infection transmitted by blood transfusion. *Transfusion* 43 (8):1018–22.

Health, C. W., and R. J. Hasterlik. 1963. Leukemia among children in a suburban community. *Am J Epidemiol* 34:796–812.

Heath, C. W., Jr., H. Falk, and J. L. Creech, Jr. 1975. Characteristics of cases of angiosarcoma of the liver among vinyl chloride workers in the United States. *Ann N Y Acad Sci* 246:231–6.

Henderson, D. A., T. V. Inglesby, J. G. Bartlett, M. S. Ascher, E. Eitzen, P. B. Jahrling, J. Hauer, M. Layton, J. McDade, M. T. Osterholm, T. O'Toole, G. Parker, T. Perl, P. K. Russell, and K. Tonat. 1999. Smallpox as a biological weapon: medical and public health management. Working Group on Civilian Biodefense. *JAMA* 281 (22):2127–37.

Hennekens, Charles H., and Julie E. Buring. 1987. *Epidemiology in medicine*. 1st ed. Boston: Little, Brown.

Holtz, T. H., J. Ackelsberg, J. L. Kool, R. Rosselli, A. Marfin, T. Matte, S. T. Beatrice, M. B. Heller, D. Hewett, L. C. Moskin, M. L. Bunning, and M. Layton. 2003. Isolated case of bioterrorism-related inhalational anthrax, New York City, 2001. *Emerg Infect Dis* 9 (6):689–96.

Holtz, T. H., et al. 2003. The public health response to the World Trade Center disaster, New York City. In *Terrorism and public health,* edited by Barry S. Levy and Victor W. Sidel. New York: Oxford University Press.

Hopkins, Donald R. 2002. *The greatest killer: smallpox in history, with a new introduction.* Chicago: University of Chicago Press.

Hsieh, Y. H., C. W. Chen, and S. B. Hsu. 2004. SARS outbreak, Taiwan, 2003. *Emerg Infect Dis* 10 (2):201–6.

Hsu, L. Y., C. C. Lee, J. A. Green, B. Ang, N. I. Paton, L. Lee, J. S. Villacian, P. L. Lim, A. Earnest, and Y. S. Leo. 2003. Severe acute respiratory syndrome (SARS) in Singapore: clinical features of index patient and initial contacts. *Emerg Infect Dis* 9 (6):713–7.

Hsu, V. P., S. L. Lukacs, T. Handzel, J. Hayslett, S. Harper, T. Hales,

V. A. Semenova, S. Romero-Steiner, C. Elie, C. P. Quinn, R. Khabbaz, A. S. Khan, G. Martin, J. Eisold, A. Schuchat, and R. A. Hajjeh. 2002. Opening a bacillus anthracis-containing envelope, Capitol Hill, Washington, DC: the public health response. *Emerg Infect Dis* 8 (10):1039–43.

Hughes, J. M., and J. L. Gerberding. 2002. Anthrax bioterrorism: lessons learned and future directions. *Emerg Infect Dis* 8 (10):1013–4.

Iwamoto, M. 2003. Transmission of West Nile virus from an organ donor to four transplant recipients—Georgia and Florida, 2002. Paper read at 52nd Annual EIS Scientific Conference, March 31–April 4, 2003, at Atlanta, Georgia.

Iwamoto, M., D. B. Jernigan, A. Guasch, M. J. Trepka, C. G. Blackmore, W. C. Hellinger, S. M. Pham, S. Zaki, R. S. Lanciotti, S. E. Lance-Parker, C. A. DiazGranados, A. G. Winquist, C. A. Perlino, S. Wiersma, K. L. Hillyer, J. L. Goodman, A. A. Marfin, M. E. Chamberland, and L. R. Petersen. 2003. Transmission of West Nile virus from an organ donor to four transplant recipients. *N Engl J Med 348* (22):2196–203.

Jereb, J., S. C. Etkind, O. T. Joglar, M. Moore, and Z. Taylor. 2003. Tuberculosis contact investigations: outcomes in selected areas of the United States, 1999. *Int J Tuberc Lung Dis* 7 (12 Suppl 3):S384–90.

Jernigan, D. B., P. L. Raghunathan, B. P. Bell, R. Brechner, E. A. Bresnitz, J. C. Butler, M. Cetron, M. Cohen, T. Doyle, M. Fischer, C. Greene, K. S. Griffith, J. Guarner, J. L. Hadler, J. A. Hayslett, R. Meyer, L. R. Petersen, M. Phillips, R. Pinner, T. Popovic, C. P. Quinn, J. Reefhuis, D. Reissman, N. Rosenstein, A. Schuchat, W. J. Shieh, L. Siegal, D. L. Swerdlow, F. C. Tenover, M. Traeger, J. W. Ward, I. Weisfuse, S. Wiersma, K. Yeskey, S. Zaki, D. A. Ashford, B. A. Perkins, S. Ostroff, J. Hughes, D. Fleming, J. P. Koplan, and J. L. Gerberding. 2002. Investigation of bioterrorism-related anthrax, United States, 2001: epidemiologic findings. *Emerg Infect Dis* 8 (10):1019–28.

Jernigan, J. A., D. S. Stephens, D. A. Ashford, C. Omenaca, M. S. Topiel, M. Galbraith, M. Tapper, T. L. Fisk, S. Zaki, T. Popovic, R. F. Meyer, C. P. Quinn, S. A. Harper, S. K. Fridkin, J. J. Sejvar, C. W. Shepard, M. McConnell, J. Guarner, W. J.

Shieh, J. M. Malecki, J. L. Gerberding, J. M. Hughes, and B. A. Perkins. 2001. Bioterrorism-related inhalational anthrax: the first 10 cases reported in the United States. *Emerg Infect Dis* 7 (6):933–44.

Johnson, L. B., A. Bhan, J. Pawlak, O. Manzor, and L. D. Saravolatz. 2003. Changing epidemiology of community-onset methicillin-resistant Staphylococcus aureus bacteremia. *Infect Control Hosp Epidemiol* 24 (6):431–5.

Keane, Fergal. 1996. *Season of blood: a Rwandan journey.* London: Penguin.

Kilbourne, E. M., J. G. Rigau-Perez, C. W. Heath, Jr., M. M. Zack, H. Falk, M. Martin-Marcos, and A. de Carlos. 1983. Clinical epidemiology of toxic-oil syndrome: manifestations of a new illness. *N Engl J Med* 309 (23):1408–14.

Koplan, J. P., and S. O. Foster. 1979. Smallpox: clinical types, causes of death, and treatment. *J Infect Dis* 140 (3):440–1.

Koplan, J. P., K. A. Monsur, S. O. Foster, F. Huq, M. M. Rahaman, S. Huq, R. A. Buchanan, and N. A. Ward. 1975. Treatment of variola major with adenine arabinoside. *J Infect Dis* 131 (1):34–9.

Koplan, J. P., and S. B. Thacker. 2001. Fifty years of epidemiology at the Centers for Disease Control and Prevention: significant and consequential. *Am J Epidemiol 154* (11):982–4.

Ksiazek, T. G., D. Erdman, C. S. Goldsmith, S. R. Zaki, T. Peret, S. Emery, S. Tong, C. Urbani, J. A. Comer, W. Lim, P. E. Rollin, S. F. Dowell, A. E. Ling, C. D. Humphrey, W. J. Shieh, J. Guarner, C. D. Paddock, P. Rota, B. Fields, J. DeRisi, J. Y. Yang, N. Cox, J. M. Hughes, J. W. LeDuc, W. J. Bellini, and L. J. Anderson. 2003. A novel coronavirus associated with severe acute respiratory syndrome. *N Engl J Med* 348 (20):1953–66.

Landrigan, P. J. 1972. Epidemic measles in a divided city. *JAMA* 221 (6):567–70.

Landrigan, P. J., E. L. Baker, Jr., R. G. Feldman, D. H. Cox, K. V. Eden, W. A. Orenstein, J. A. Mather, A. J. Yankel, and I. H. Von Lindern. 1976. Increased lead absorption with anemia and slowed nerve conduction in children near a lead smelter. *J Pediatr* 89 (6):904–10.

Landrigan, P. J., S. H. Gehlbach, B. F. Rosenblum, J. M. Shoults, R. M. Candelaria, W. F. Barthel, J. A. Liddle, A. L. Smrek, N. W. Staehling, and J. F. Sanders. 1975. Epidemic lead absorption near an ore smelter: the role of particulate lead. *N Engl J Med* 292 (3):123–9.

Landrigan, P. J., R. H. Whitworth, R. W. Baloh, N. W. Staehling, W. F. Barthel, and B. F. Rosenblum. 1975. Neuropsychological dysfunction in children with chronic low-level lead absorption. *Lancet* 1 (7909):708–12.

Lane, J. M. 2002. Smallpox and smallpox vaccination. *N Engl J Med* 347 (9):691–2.

Lane, J. M., F. L. Ruben, J. M. Neff, and J. D. Millar. 1969. Complications of smallpox vaccination, 1968. *N Engl J Med* 281 (22):1201–8.

———. 1970. Complications of smallpox vaccination, 1968: results of ten statewide surveys. *J Infect Dis* 122 (4):303–9.

Langmuir, A. D. 1951. The potentialities of biological warfare against man: an epidemiological appraisal. *Public Health Rep* 66 (13):387–99.

———. 1980. The Epidemic Intelligence Service of the Center for Disease Control. *Public Health Rep* 95 (5):470–7.

Langmuir, A. D., and J. M. Andrews. 1952. Biological warfare defense. 2. The Epidemic Intelligence Service of the Communicable Disease Center. *Am J Public Health* 42 (3):235–8.

Lau, J. T., K. S. Fung, T. W. Wong, J. H. Kim, E. Wong, S. Chung, D. Ho, L. Y. Chan, S. F. Lui, and A. Cheng. 2004. SARS transmission among hospital workers in Hong Kong. *Emerg Infect Dis* 10 (2):280–6.

Le, D. H., S. A. Bloom, Q. H. Nguyen, S. A. Maloney, Q. M. Le, K. C. Leitmeyer, H. A. Bach, M. G. Reynolds, J. M. Montgomery, J. A. Comer, P. W. Horby, and A. J. Plant. 2004. Lack of SARS transmission among public hospital workers, Vietnam. *Emerg Infect Dis* 10 (2):265–8.

Leavitt, J. W. 2003. Public resistance or cooperation? A tale of smallpox in two cities. *Biosecur Bioterror* 1 (3):185–92.

Lederberg, Joshua, Robert E. Shope, and Stanley C. Oaks Jr., eds. 1992. *Emerging infections: microbial threats to health in the*

United States. Washington, DC: Institute of Medicine, National Academy of Sciences, National Academies Press.

Lee, N., D. Hui, A. Wu, P. Chan, P. Cameron, G. M. Joynt, A. Ahuja, M. Y. Yung, C. B. Leung, K. F. To, S. F. Lui, C. C. Szeto, S. Chung, and J. J. Sung. 2003. A major outbreak of severe acute respiratory syndrome in Hong Kong. *N Engl J Med* 348 (20):1986–94.

Macaulay, Thomas Babington Macaulay, and C. H. Firth. 1913. *The history of England, from the accession of James the Second*. London: Macmillan.

Marfin, A. A., L. R. Petersen, M. Eidson, J. Miller, J. Hadler, C. Farello, B. Werner, G. L. Campbell, M. Layton, P. Smith, E. Bresnitz, M. Cartter, J. Scaletta, G. Obiri, M. Bunning, R. C. Craven, J. T. Roehrig, K. G. Julian, S. R. Hinten, and D. J. Gubler. 2001. Widespread West Nile virus activity, eastern United States, 2000. *Emerg Infect Dis* 7 (4):730–5.

Masur, H., M. A. Michelis, J. B. Greene, I. Onorato, R. A. Stouwe, R. S. Holzman, G. Wormser, L. Brettman, M. Lange, H. W. Murray, and S. Cunningham-Rundles. 1981. An outbreak of community-acquired Pneumocystis carinii pneumonia: initial manifestation of cellular immune dysfunction. *N Engl J Med* 305 (24):1431–8.

McElroy, P. D., R. B. Rothenberg, R. Varghese, R. Woodruff, G. O. Minns, S. Q. Muth, L. A. Lambert, and R. Ridzon. 2003. A network-informed approach to investigating a tuberculosis outbreak: implications for enhancing contact investigations. *Int J Tuberc Lung Dis* 7 (12 Suppl 3):S486–93.

McElroy, P. D., K. L. Southwick, E. R. Fortenberry, E. C. Levine, L. A. Diem, C. L. Woodley, P. M. Williams, K. D. McCarthy, R. Ridzon, and P. A. Leone. 2003. Outbreak of tuberculosis among homeless persons coinfected with human immunodeficiency virus. *Clin Infect Dis* 36 (10):1305–12.

McElroy, P. D., T. R. Sterling, C. R. Driver, B. Kreiswirth, C. L. Woodley, W. A. Cronin, D. X. Hardge, K. L. Shilkret, and R. Ridzon. 2002. Use of DNA fingerprinting to investigate a multiyear, multistate tuberculosis outbreak. *Emerg Infect Dis* 8 (11):1252–6.

McNeill, William Hardy. 1998. *Plagues and peoples.* New York: Anchor Books/Doubleday.

McNinch, J. H. 1953. Far East Command Conference on Epidemic Hemorrhagic Fever; introduction. *Ann Intern Med* 38 (1):53–60.

Mead, P. S., L. Slutsker, V. Dietz, L. F. McCaig, J. S. Bresee, C. Shapiro, P. M. Griffin, and R. V. Tauxe. 1999. Food-related illness and death in the United States. *Emerg Infect Dis* 5 (5):607–25.

Monsur, K. A., M. S. Hossain, F. Huq, M. M. Rahaman, and M. Q. Haque. 1975. Treatment of variola major with cytosine arabinoside. *J Infect Dis* 131 (1):40–3.

Montgomery, S. 2004. Screening of the National Blood Supply for West Nile Virus—United States, 2003. Paper read at Fifth National Conference on West Nile Virus in the United States, Feb. 3–5, 2004, at Denver, Colorado.

Mullan, Fitzhugh. 1989. *Plagues and politics: the story of the United States Public Health Service.* New York: Basic Books.

Nathanson, N., and E. R. Alexander. 1996. Infectious disease epidemiology. *Am J Epidemiol* 144 (8 Suppl):S34–8.

Nathanson, N., and A. D. Langmuir. 1963. The Cutter incident: Poliomyelitis following formaldehyde-inactivated poliovirus vaccination in the United States during the spring of 1955. I. Background. *Am J Hyg* 78:16–28.

———. 1963. The Cutter incident: Poliomyelitis following formaldehyde-inactivated poliovirus vaccination in the United States during the spring of 1955. II. Relationship of poliomyelitis to Cutter vaccine. *Am J Hyg* 78:29–60.

———. 1963. The Cutter incident: poliomyelitis following formaldehyde-inactivated poliovirus vaccination in the United States during the spring of 1955. III. Comparison of the clinical character of vaccinated and contact cases occurring after use of high rate lots of Cutter vaccine. *Am J Hyg* 78: 61–81.

Neff, J. M., J. M. Lane, and V. A. Fulginiti. 2003. Smallpox and smallpox vaccination. *N Engl J Med* 348 (19):1920–5.

Newbern, Claire. 2003. Multi-State Listeriosis Outbreak Associated with Turkey Deli Meat, 2002. Paper read at Council of State and Territorial Epidemiologists annual meeting, June 22–26, 2003, at Hartford, Conn.

Oakley, G. P., Jr., and C. W. Heath, Jr. 1996. Cancer, environmental health, and birth defects—examples of new directions in public health practice. *Am J Epidemiol* 144 (8 Suppl):S58–64.

Ogden, Horace G., and Centers for Disease Control (U.S.). 1987. *CDC and the smallpox crusade.* Washington, DC: U.S. Dept. of Health and Human Services, Public Health Service.

Ostroff, S. M. 2001. Le Service d'Investigation Epidemique aux Etats-Unis. *Euro Surveill* 6 (3):34–6.

Payer, Lynn. 1996. *Medicine and culture: varieties of treatment in the United States, England, West Germany, and France.* First Owl Book ed. New York: Henry Holt.

Perkins, B. A., T. Popovic, and K. Yeskey. 2002. Public health in the time of bioterrorism. *Emerg Infect Dis* 8 (10):1015–8.

Peters, C. J., and Mark Olshaker. 1997. *Virus hunter: Thirty years of battling hot viruses around the world.* New York: Anchor Books.

Petersen, L. R., and J. T. Roehrig. 2001. West Nile virus: a reemerging global pathogen. *Emerg Infect Dis* 7 (4):611–4.

Plotkin, Stanley A., and Walter A. Orenstein. 1999. *Vaccines.* 3rd ed. Philadelphia: W. B. Saunders.

Poutanen, S. M., D. E. Low, B. Henry, S. Finkelstein, D. Rose, K. Green, R. Tellier, R. Draker, D. Adachi, M. Ayers, A. K. Chan, D. M. Skowronski, I. Salit, A. E. Simor, A. S. Slutsky, P. W. Doyle, M. Krajden, M. Petric, R. C. Brunham, and A. J. McGeer. 2003. Identification of severe acute respiratory syndrome in Canada. *N Engl J Med* 348 (20):1995–2005.

Preston, Richard. 2002. *The demon in the freezer: a true story.* New York: Random House.

ProMED-mail. 2003. *Pneumonia—China (Guangdong) (02). 11 Feb:* 20030211.0369 2003 [cited 2003]. Available from www.promedmail.org.

———. 2003. *Pneumonia—China (Guangdong) (03). 14 Feb:* 20030214.0390 2003 [cited 2003]. Available from www.promedmail.org.

———. 2003. *Pneumonia—China (Guangdong) (04). 19 Feb:* 20030219.0427 2003 [cited 2003]. Available from www.promedmail.org.

————. 2003. *Pneumonia—China (Guangdong) (06)*. 20 Feb: 20030220.0447 2003 [cited 2003]. Available from www.promedmail.org.

————. 2003. *Pneumonia—China (Guangdong): RFI*. 10 Feb: 20030210.0357 2003 [cited 2003]. Available from www.promedmail.org.

Ravenholt, Reimert. 2003. *Becoming an epidemiologist* [cited 2003]. Available from www.ravenholt.com.

Reingold, A.L. 2001. Perspectives prometteuses pour la formation en épidemiologie de terrain en Europe. *Euro Surveill* 6 (3):33–4.

Reiter, P. 2000. From Shakespeare to Defoe: malaria in England in the Little Ice Age. *Emerg Infect Dis* 6 (1):1–11.

Rigau-Perez, JG. 2001. The Toxic Oil Syndrome in Spain, 1981. Paper read at 50th Annual EIS Scientific Conference, at Atlanta, Georgia.

Roberts, L., and M. J. Toole. 1995. Cholera deaths in Goma. *Lancet* 346 (8987):1431.

Roehrig, J. T., D. Nash, B. Maldin, A. Labowitz, D. A. Martin, R. S. Lanciotti, and G. L. Campbell. 2003. Persistence of virus-reactive serum immunoglobulin m antibody in confirmed West Nile virus encephalitis cases. *Emerg Infect Dis* 9 (3):376–9.

Rogers, Naomi. 1992. *Dirt and disease: polio before FDR. Health and medicine in American society*. New Brunswick, NJ: Rutgers University Press.

————. 1997. Dirt, flies and immigrants: explaining the epidemiology of poliomyelitis, 1900–1916. In *Sickness and health in America*, edited by Judith Waltzer Leavitt and Ronald L. Numbers. Madison: University of Wisconsin Press.

Rosenberg, Charles E. 1997. Framing disease: illness, society and history. In *Framing disease: studies in cultural history*, edited by Charles E. Rosenberg and Janet Golden. New Brunswick, NJ: Rutgers University Press.

Roueche, Berton. 1991. *The medical detectives*. New York: Truman Talley Books/Plume.

Ruane, P. et al. 2003. Outbreak of Clonal Methicillin Resistant Staphylococcus Infection in an Outpatient Infectious Disease Practice in Los Angeles. Poster presented at Second Conference of the International AIDS Society: Pathogenesis and Treatment of HIV, July 13–16, 2003, Paris.

Said-Salim, B., B. Mathema, and B. N. Kreiswirth. 2003. Community-acquired methicillin-resistant Staphylococcus aureus: an emerging pathogen. *Infect Control Hosp Epidemiol* 24 (6):451–5.

Schaffner, W., and F. M. LaForce. 1996. Training field epidemiologists: Alexander D. Langmuir and the epidemic intelligence service. *Am J Epidemiol* 144 (8 Suppl):S16–22.

Schmaljohn, C., and B. Hjelle. 1997. Hantaviruses: a global disease problem. *Emerg Infect Dis* 3 (2):95–104.

Schnabel, James F. UNITED STATES ARMY IN THE KOREAN WAR: Policy and direction, the first year. CENTER OF MILITARY HISTORY, UNITED STATES ARMY [cited 2003.] Available from www.army.mil/cmh-pg/books/P&d.htm.

Sepkowitz, K. A. 2003. How contagious is vaccinia? *N Engl J Med* 348 (5):439–46.

Shen, Z., F. Ning, W. Zhou, X. He, C. Lin, D. P. Chin, Z. Zhu, and A. Schuchat. 2004. Superspreading SARS events, Beijing, 2003. *Emerg Infect Dis* 10 (2):256–60.

Shilts, Randy. 1987. *And the band played on: politics, people, and the AIDS epidemic.* New York: St. Martin's Press.

Smith, Jane S. 1990. *Patenting the sun: polio and the Salk vaccine.* New York: W. Morrow.

Smolinski, Mark S., Margaret A. Hamburg, and Joshua Lederberg, eds. 2003. *Microbial threats to health: emergence, detection, and response.* Washington, DC: Institute of Medicine, National Academy of Science, National Academies Press.

Sterling, T. R., D. Thompson, R. L. Stanley, P. D. McElroy, A. Madison, K. Moore, R. Ridzon, S. Harrington, W. R. Bishai, R. E. Chaisson, and S. Bur. 2000. A multi-state outbreak of tuberculosis among members of a highly mobile social network: implications for tuberculosis elimination. *Int J Tuberc Lung Dis* 4 (11):1066–73.

Strommen, Catherine. 2003 Teachers.Net Chatroom Exchange Reveals SARS Outbreak. Teachers.Net Gazette, Vol. 4 No. 6

[cited 2003.] Available from http://teachers.net/gazette/JUN03/strommen.html.

Swaminathan, B., T. J. Barrett, S. B. Hunter, and R. V. Tauxe. 2001. PulseNet: the molecular subtyping network for foodborne bacterial disease surveillance, United States. *Emerg Infect Dis* 7 (3):382–9.

Swerdlow, D. L., O. Levine, M. J. Toole, R. J. Waldman, and R. V. Tauxe. 1994. Cholera control among Rwandan refugees in Zaire. *Lancet* 344 (8932):1302–3.

Tabuenca, J. M. 1981. Toxic-allergic syndrome caused by ingestion of rapeseed oil denatured with aniline. *Lancet* 2 (8246):567–8.

Tauxe, R. V. 2001. My life in medicine: practicing the science of epidemiology and the art of public health. *Infect Dis in Clin Prac* 10:241–8.

Thacker, S. B., and J. Buffington. 2001. Applied epidemiology for the 21st century. *Int J Epidemiol* 30 (2):320–5.

Thacker, S. B., A. L. Dannenberg, and D. H. Hamilton. 2001. Epidemic intelligence service of the Centers for Disease Control and Prevention: 50 years of training and service in applied epidemiology. *Am J Epidemiol* 154 (11):985–92.

Thacker, S. B., R. A. Goodman, and R. C. Dicker. 1990. Training and service in public health practice, 1951–90—CDC's Epidemic Intelligence Service. *Public Health Rep* 105 (6):599–604.

Thacker, S. B., and M. B. Gregg. 1996. Implementing the concepts of William Farr: the contributions of Alexander D. Langmuir to public health surveillance and communications. *Am J Epidemiol* 144 (8 Suppl):S23–8.

Thomas, Gordon, and Max Morgan Witts. 1982. *Anatomy of an epidemic.* Garden City, NY: Doubleday.

Thomas, Patricia. 2003. *The anthrax attacks.* New York: Century Foundation.

Thompson, Marilyn W. 2003. *The killer strain: anthrax and a government exposed.* New York: HarperCollins.

Traeger, M. S., S. T. Wiersma, N. E. Rosenstein, J. M. Malecki, C. W. Shepard, P. L. Raghunathan, S. P. Pillai, T. Popovic, C. P. Quinn, R. F. Meyer, S. R. Zaki, S. Kumar, S. M. Bruce, J. J. Sejvar, P. M. Dull, B. C. Tierney, J. D. Jones, and B. A. Perkins. 2002. First case of bioterrorism-related inhalational anthrax in the United States, Palm Beach County, Florida, 2001. *Emerg Infect Dis* 8 (10):1029–34.

Tsang, K. W., P. L. Ho, G. C. Ooi, W. K. Yee, T. Wang, M. Chan-Yeung, W. K. Lam, W. H. Seto, L. Y. Yam, T. M. Cheung, P. C. Wong, B. Lam, M. S. Ip, J. Chan, K. Y. Yuen, and K. N. Lai. 2003. A cluster of cases of severe acute respiratory syndrome in Hong Kong. *N Engl J Med* 348 (20):1977–85.

Tucker, Jonathan B. 2001. *Scourge: the once and future threat of smallpox.* New York: Atlantic Monthly Press.

Van Damme, W. 1995. Do refugees belong in camps? Experiences from Goma and Guinea. *Lancet* 346 (8971):360–2.

Vu, H. T., K. C. Leitmeyer, D. H. Le, M. J. Miller, Q. H. Nguyen, T. M. Uyeki, M. G. Reynolds, J. Aagesen, K. G. Nicholson, Q. H. Vu, H. A. Bach, and A. J. Plan. 2004. Clinical description of a completed outbreak of SARS in Vietnam, February–May 2003. *Emerg Infect Dis* 10 (2):334–8.

Wills, Christopher. 1996. *Yellow fever, black goddess: the coevolution of people and plagues.* Reading, MA: Addison-Wesley.

Wong, R. S., and D. S. Hui. 2004. Index patient and SARS outbreak in Hong Kong. *Emerg Infect Dis* 10 (2):339–41.

Wong, T. W., C. K. Lee, W. Tam, J. T. Lau, T. S. Yu, S. F. Lui, P. K. Chan, Y. Li, J. S. Bresee, J. J. Sung, and U. D. Parashar. 2004. Cluster of SARS among medical students exposed to single patient, Hong Kong. *Emerg Infect Dis* 10 (2):269–76.

World Health Organization. Global Commission for the Certification of Smallpox Eradication. 1980. *The global eradication of smallpox: final report of the Global Commission for the Certification of Smallpox Eradication, Geneva, December 1979. History of international public health; no. 4.* Geneva: World Health Organization, WHO Publications Centre.

Zinsser, Hans. 1935. *Rats, lice and history; being a study in biography, which, after twelve preliminary chapters indispensable for the preparation of the lay reader, deals with the life history of typhus fever.* Boston: Printed for the Atlantic Monthly Press by Little, Brown.

ACKNOWLEDGMENTS

This book would not exist were it not for the many members of the Epidemic Intelligence Service and other veterans of the Centers for Disease Control and Prevention who shared their time, their records and their inexhaustible funds of stories. Particular thanks are due to J. Lyle Conrad, William H. Foege, Jeffrey P. Koplan, J. Michael Lane and David J. Sencer. I also thank Philip S. Brachman and Alan R. Hinman of the EIS Alumni Association for assisting me in my research.

At the CDC, Stephen B. Thacker, Douglas H. Hamilton and Jim Alexander of the CDC's Epidemiology Program Office were unfailingly generous with documents and explanations. Laura Fehrs of that office, Ross Cox in Global Health and Donald J. Sharp in Food Safety opened doors that would otherwise have been closed to me. Kathryn Harben of the Office of Communications was a good-humored, professional and exceptionally patient guide through the intricacies of the CDC. Lisa Swenarski, now with the State Department, was an early champion of this project. I am grateful to them all.

Outside the CDC's campuses, I received extraordinary assistance from many people who are or were affiliated with the agency. Thank you to James W. Buehler of the Georgia Division of Public Health, Scott F. Wetterhall of the DeKalb County Board of Health, and C. Charles Stokes, Linda Kane, and Linda Kay McGowan of the CDC Foundation in Atlanta, as well as Rick Schlegel of the Center for Domestic Preparedness in Anniston, Alabama. In Bangkok, I owe great debts to Scott and Robin Dowell and Mike Martin and Rachel Rodriguez. I could not have navigated through Hanoi without the help of Mary Kamb and Michael J. Linnan, or found my way in Malawi without the hospitality of Carl and Joy Campbell. Thanks are due also to Paul Simon, Laurene Mascola and Frank Sorvillo in Los Angeles and Thomas J. Safranek in Nebraska.

Michael T. Osterholm of the University of Minnesota knows the CDC better than many who have worked there, and his insights into its concerns and culture were always apposite and worthwhile.

At the Free Press, I am grateful to my editor, Elizabeth Stein, for her insight, sympathy and support, and to her assistants Maris Kreizman and Stephanie Fairyington. I value the welcome extended to me by Free Press publisher Martha Levin and editorial director Dominick Anfuso.

I am quite sure I do not deserve the creativity, tenacity and acumen of my agent, Susan Raihofer, but I am grateful to benefit from them. Thank you also to her assistant Leigh Ann Eliseo, and to my former colleague Gary M. Pomerantz, who effected my introduction to the David Black Literary Agency.

This book had its genesis in stories I wrote about the EIS for the *Atlanta Journal-Constitution* and would not have been possible without the support of my editors and colleagues. I particularly thank Julia Wallace, Hank Klibanoff, Susan Stevenson, Barb Senftleber, Arthur Brice, Nancy Albritton and David Wahlberg.

While reporting and writing, I received excellent and essential help from Michele Powell of National Quality Transcripts Inc. and Donna Grace of Grace Executive Services, and their respective staffs of rapid, reliable, accurate transcriptionists; and from Patricia Hynes, Alice Wertheim, Steven Ashby, Carol Grizzle and Susana Francesconi.

Many friends and family fed, housed and otherwise helped me in many locations, and I am grateful to all of them: Samara Cummins, Rich Eldredge and Krista Reese in Atlanta; Paul Levitt in Boston; Wayne Turnbull in Hanoi; John McKenna in Houston; Wayne and Nancy Casper in Lincoln; Matt McKenna and Darla Albright in Los Angeles; Melynda Forsythe in Minneapolis; Father Robert E. Lauder and Lisa Jones in New York; Nancy Cooney in Philadelphia; and Bob McKenna and Cerise McKenna Vablais in Washington, DC.

Last and best I thank Loren Dewey Bolstridge III. Without his warmth, wit, affection and as-yet unflagging support, none of this would have been possible, or worthwhile.

INDEX

ABOUT THE AUTHOR

MARYN MCKENNA is an award-winning science and medical writer at the *Atlanta Journal-Constitution,* where she has covered the CDC since 1997. She is a graduate of Georgetown University and the Medill School of Journalism at Northwestern University and has also studied at Harvard Medical School. In 1998–1999 she was the Knight Fellow in Medicine at the University of Michigan's schools of medicine and public health. She lives in Atlanta.